Low intensity support services

A systematic literature review

Deborah Quilgars

The **POLICY**

P P

P R E S S

First published in Great Britain in ~~July 2000 by~~

The Policy Press
34 Tyndall's Park Road
Bristol BS8 1PY
UK

Tel no +44 (0)117 954 6800
Fax no +44 (0)117 973 7308
E-mail tpp@bristol.ac.uk
www.policypress.org.uk

Published for the Joseph Rowntree Foundation by The Policy Press

ISBN 1 86134 239 X

Deborah Quilgars is a Research Fellow at the Centre for Housing Policy, University of York.

The **Joseph Rowntree Foundation** has supported this project as part of its programme of research and innovative development projects, which it hopes will be of value to policy makers, practitioners and service users. The facts presented and views expressed in this report are, however, those of the authors and not necessarily those of the Foundation.

Cover design by Qube Design Associates, Bristol
Printed in Great Britain by Hobbs the Printers Ltd, Southampton

Contents

Acknowledgements

My sincere thanks go to the members of the Joseph Rowntree Foundation Advisory Group for their helpful advice and assistance throughout the project: Heather Clark, Mary Taylor, Ken Simons, John Lockhart and Mike Coates. I am also very grateful to Alison Jarvis for her constant support and patience, and to Janet Lewis for suggesting the idea of a review in this area.

I would not have been able to undertake the review without the expert skills of Lisa Mather, Information Officer in the NHS Centre for Reviews and Dissemination at the University of York, who undertook all the database searches.

Finally, my thanks also go to Jane Allen and Lynne Lonsdale for preparing the manuscript at breakneck speed.

Introduction

This report presents the findings of a systematic literature review examining the effectiveness of low intensity support services, used to enable people in need of support to live independently in their own homes. This chapter begins by examining the policy background which informs, and provides the rationale for undertaking a systematic review in this area.

The 1990s: community care and the emphasis on high intensity care

It is now widely accepted that, over the past decade, limited statutory community care resources have been increasingly targeted on high level need – often crisis interventions – at the expense of prioritising lower level, preventative services (Audit Commission, 1998; Joseph Rowntree Foundation, 1999).

The home care service may provide the best example of increased targeting of services. By the late 1980s home 'help' services had started the transformation from a primarily domestic service to one with a greater emphasis on personal 'care' (Sinclair and Williams, 1990). This process was accelerated by the introduction of the community care reforms, with services being increasingly targeted at those in greatest need of home support away from a wider coverage of less intensive services (SSI, 1993; Audit Commission, 1996). Department of Health (DoH) statistics on local authority-funded home care show that the average number of contact hours per person increased from 3.2 hours in 1992 to 5.5 hours in 1997 (DoH, 1997a, 1997b), while there has been a slight reduction in the number of households receiving the service overall (DoH, 1997a). While most people receiving home care services are aged over 65, younger client groups – such as people with physical and/or sensory disabilities – tend to be allocated a higher amount of funded care per person than is the case for older people (Hall, 1997). While there has always been variability between local authorities, and about a quarter of home care users still only receive one visit a week, in the mid-1990s the Audit Commission (1996) suggested that those authorities providing a low number of hours to a large number of people might need to consider increasingly targeting the service.

Increased targeting has also occurred within the mental health field. There has been a concern that while reprovision arrangements to resettle long-stay patients from the former psychiatric institutions have generally been successful (House of Commons Health Committee, 1994), replacement health and social services community facilities have not been adequate to meet the continuing needs of people with mental health problems. In particular there is concern for people who suffer long-term mental health problems, who may have spent large periods of their life in an institution but now live in the community. Health and social services support services are increasingly focused on providing crisis interventions for people presenting acute or high level needs, and are rarely able to provide services to people who, at the time, are exhibiting lower level needs. This too often results in the 'revolving door' problem of people's health being at a heightened risk of deteriorating to the point at which they need crisis interventions and a hospital admission, instead of any problems being identified and managed through the continued input of a low level of support. This "all or nothing" system (Audit Commission, 1998) can be costly to both the individual and the organisations involved.

Services for people with learning difficulties and physical impairments have been similarly focused on high intensity needs. Reprovision arrangements and more general developments for people with learning difficulties have predominantly consisted of permanent supported residential or shared group homes, almost to the total exclusion of independent living arrangements (Simons, 1997). Similarly, where services have been developed for disabled people, the focus has often been on the provision of specialist schemes (Esmond and Stewart, 1997), and although the importance of high level personal assistance schemes to support people in their own homes has been increasingly recognised (Kestenbaum, 1996), lower level services continue to receive less attention.

Increasing low intensity support needs

While statistics are elusive, and residential and specialist schemes still dominate provision, it is generally accepted that changes in community care policy, combined with wider socioeconomic forces, has led to an increasing proportion of people with support needs living in ordinary tenancies in the 'community', usually alone and often unsupported. In particular, there is now considerable evidence which indicates that economically marginalised households, including people with community care and support needs, are becoming relatively concentrated in the social rented sector. New households entering social housing in the early to mid-1990s were significantly more likely to be unemployed, to be younger (including lone parents) and to be members of ethnic minorities than existing tenants (Burrows, 1997). Only 26% of new households were in full-time employment, with 31% unemployed and 34% being unable to work (not including retired people). Another study estimated that a majority of new tenants housed in general needs accommodation by registered social landlords (RSLs) in London could be considered 'vulnerable' in some way (London Housing Federation, 1995). Further, those not fortunate enough to gain access to the social rented sector have to rely on the often poor quality lower end of the private rented sector, or indeed may face homelessness.

There has been considerable concern about the lack of support available to tenants with support needs in general needs housing. Unsupported, people may experience problems in maintaining their independence and their health. A number of reports have suggested that tenancies are more likely to break down (Hammond and Wallace, 1992; Pleace, 1995), costing local authorities around £2,000 a time in unrecoverable arrears, redecoration and cleaning costs, repairs, staff time and subsequent homelessness application (Audit Commission, 1998). A number of reports (London Housing Federation, 1995, 1997; Pettitt and Frew, 1998) have focused on the need for better interagency working, and ways of improving the information and assessment systems to firstly, identify, and secondly, address the support needs of 'vulnerable' tenants. Studies have unsurprisingly shown that housing managers feel both unqualified and lacking in resources to address many of these issues (Clapham and Franklin, 1995). There have also been widespread doubts as to whether the provision of support is compatible with increasing commercial pressures on the core business of a social landlord, particularly compulsory competitive tendering (Clapham and Franklin, 1995; Pettitt and Frew, 1998).

Notwithstanding this, many housing authorities and RSLs have tried, often with very limited resources, to support an increasingly socially marginalised and/or 'vulnerable' tenant population. These issues go right to the centre of well-rehearsed debates about the role and definition of housing services, housing management, intensive housing management and support (as well as, of course, the definitional boundaries between support and care). For example, even at its most basic, there does not appear to be a consensus on how to draw the boundary of housing management (Lesley Andrews, 1998). The management of social housing has always extended beyond property management in some way, what has sometimes been referred to as the 'welfare' role or, simply, 'social' role of housing (Clapham and Franklin, 1994). However, the definitional clarity of this role has always been elusive: it has been clearer what the welfare role is *not* (ie the provision of personal social services and health services – particularly 'personal care') than what the welfare role actually *is*. Basic housing management is perhaps the simplest area to define as it encompasses the main landlord functions of allocations, collecting rents, repairs and so on. Intensive housing management encompasses similar tasks but are generally more intensively delivered to people who may require some guidance on conditions of tenancy, welfare benefits and so on to enable them to perform their duties as a tenant. Further to this, tenancy support may encompass both practical, housing and non-housing related tasks, for example, including assistance with moving and settling into the tenancy and emotional/ social support.

In contrast, those people with support needs living in the private rented sector are even less likely to have access to basic tenancy support services, given the present tenure specificity of local authority and Housing Corporation funding. Those with support needs in owner-occupation, most particularly older people who are 'capital-rich' but 'income poor', may have similar problems accessing general support. Here, homeowners are likely to be reliant on qualifying for home support services or voluntary sector initiatives which may be more available in some areas than others.

Present policy: a renewed emphasis on low intensity support?

A number of initiatives and policy developments over the last two years have begun to reassert the importance of the value of low level support services.

The publication of the Department of Social Security (DSS) consultation paper *Supporting people* at the end of 1998 (DSS, 1998) focused attention on the supported housing sector and the central role of preventative and low level housing services. The main objectives of the support services identified under *Supporting people* are seen as: prevention, promoting independence, alleviating crises, resettlement and inclusion. The consultation paper recognised a number of problem areas within the existing system for funding housing and support, most of which the housing world and academics had long championed for change. These areas include the complexity and piecemeal nature of funding (Clapham and Franklin, 1994); the tenure specificity of most sources of funding; and work disincentives, especially when support services are funded via the Housing Benefit system. The paper also acknowledged the limitations of offering housing and support together as a package rather than separately, so that support can be tailored to the needs of an individual (Simons, 1999), and can float in and out as required (as with The Housing Corporation Supported Housing Management Grant). For the government, however, there was also a concern at an increasing Housing Benefit bill, similar to the problems with the DSS budget for residential care pre-1993. However, a proposed shift from a needs-led to cash-limited system has been met with concern by the housing movement, as this may lead to future expansion of support services being more difficult than under a needs-led system.

Following the responses to the consultation process, which were generally favourable (although a number of reservations were expressed on the details of the implementation), the government announced in March 1999 that they would proceed with the main elements of the proposed system. From 2003, a new specific grant will be allocated to local authorities with money from the previous main funding sources (primarily Housing Benefit and The Housing Corporation Supported Housing Management Grant). Commissioning panels set up by the local authorities, involving all key agencies, will assess local support needs and commission services. Importantly, the new grant will be paid to fund services independent of the provision of accommodation or linked to it, so that support services will be just as easily provided to homeowners as to tenants. From April 2000 a transitional system will operate to begin the process of quantifying the present levels of provision through the Housing Benefit system.

In the personal social services, the recent White Paper, *Modernising social services* (DoH, 1998a), announced a new Prevention Grant of £100 million over three years to stimulate the development of preventative strategies and to target low level support services for "people most at risk of losing their independence". The local authority guidance (LAC(99)14) advised authorities to consider how they could screen people who would benefit from preventative services *into* low intensity preventative services rather than screening them *out* of high intensity services. Prevention is defined in the guidance as "action intended to prevent or delay loss of independence and to improve quality of life". The threshold for 'non-intensive' services is actually quite high: services must not exceed 10 hours per week on aggregate or more than six visits a week, therefore the impact of this grant on very low intensity services will depend on how the grant is targeted. The grant is available for a range of services and for all user groups, although the recent report by the Social Services Inspectorate (SSI, 1999) on preventative strategies for older people perhaps indicates that older people, who are numerically the largest group of people requiring support, are expected to be the main beneficiaries of the new grant.

A number of developments in the health field are also relevant to the development of low intensity support services. The White Paper, *The new NHS* (DoH, 1997c), places an onus on health authorities to produce Health Improvement Programmes, and outlines the new responsibilities of Primary Care Groups to promote health. This provides a clear indication of the current policy concern about health promotion within local communities. The public health Green Paper, *Our healthier nation* (DoH, 1998b), has also stressed the need for a preventative philosophy in addressing public health – identifying Healthy Neighbourhoods as one of its main foci. Health Action Zones, with their close link to the Green Paper, are also being used as a new method of tackling health inequalities at a local level.

Emphasis on service outcome measurements

While the value of the preventative and sustaining role of low level services is finding its way back onto the policy agenda, this has, in great part, arisen against a backdrop of poor quality data measuring the success of support services in meeting their aims. This, again, is possibly set to change as increasing pressure from a number of directions is heightening the impetus for the development of better methods of assessing service provision.

For example, the National Housing Federation (NHF) has put together *A framework for housing with support: A tool to describe, evaluate and continuously improve services* (Goss, 1998), building on the existing NHF Housing, Care and Support Code. Standards are put forward on individual rights/care, support/organisation and management/staffing; training and volunteers/physical environment/services provided. The document notes the debates about the balance between measures of service provision: *inputs* (for example, staffing levels, funding); *process standards* (for example, quality of intervention, management); *outputs* (for example, productivity, service volume) and *outcomes* (for example, impact on users' lives, user satisfaction). They also note the lack of attention on both outputs and outcomes in the past.

The clearest impetus for change comes directly from the government. In particular, the government's new Best Value framework, along with the Audit Commission's related performance indicators, have established a system by which providers of public services (including housing and social services) are asked to demonstrate Best Value in services, in terms of delivering efficient and effective services to meet a range of pre-identified measures. However, while these indicators may be useful in some areas and do take account of user satisfaction issues, they may not be sensitive enough to evaluate the effectiveness of low level support services.

The *Supporting people* document (DSS, 1998) noted the importance of local authorities using both the Best Value framework and the National Housing Federation *Framework for housing with support* to manage the new system effectively and to ensure that quality issues are adequately addressed. The *Supporting people* initiative and the introduction of the DoH Prevention Grant both provide opportunities for improving the monitoring of low level support services. However, government support, including the funding of further research into measuring outcomes, will be essential to this process.

The study

The discussion on low level support services has taken place largely without a systematic and comprehensive assessment of the evidence of the role of low intensity support services. This project sought to inform the debate through the completion of a systematic literature review of the effectiveness of such services. The overall aim of the project is to provide information which will be useful in the development of the most appropriate low level services.

The report is presented in six chapters. As the method of systematic reviewing is relatively new to social policy, Chapter 2 provides a description of the review method; it is hoped that this may be useful for other social scientists interested in conducting evidence-based reviews. Chapters 3, 4 and 5 present the main findings of the review: Chapter 3 focuses on tenancy or housing support services which enable people to establish and maintain independent accommodation themselves; Chapter 4 considers the value of practical services which are undertaken on behalf of people with support needs; Chapter 5 focuses on the importance of services which aim to increase people's social links and/or provide companionship or befriending. The final chapter presents the conclusions from the study.

2

The review: scope and methods

This chapter outlines the methods involved in undertaking the review of low intensity support services. The method of systematic reviewing is introduced and the problems with applying this methodology to social policy are discussed. The chapter then outlines the main stages involved in the review, beginning with the task of defining the scope of the study, the process followed for the literature search, the selection of studies to be included in the review and, lastly, assessment of the research evidence.

Undertaking a systematic review: the method

Evidence-based systematic reviews – originally developed in the education field – are most commonly used for assessing the benefits of health interventions. However, the systematic review process remains largely untested within the field of social policy study. While literature reviewing, more generally, has always been a staple ingredient of social policy research, there is no tradition of using standard approaches to summarise and assess research evidence as there is in systematic reviewing. Nonetheless, there is a growing interest in this method and it is a developing expertise among social policy researchers. For example, the Economic and Social

Research Council (ESRC) – the main funder of social
science research in the UK – has recently embarked on a
programme of evidence-based policy and practice
research, and is currently funding the University of York to
carry out a pilot study investigating methodologies for
conducting systematic reviews in social policy. This
methodology is likely to grow in importance in future
years.

A systematic review has been defined by the University of
York NHS Centre for Reviews and Dissemination as:

> ... the process of systematically locating,
> appraising and synthesising evidence from
> scientific studies in order to obtain a reliable
> overview. (Deeks et al, 1996)

Immediately, this definition raises questions about the
applicability of the method to social policy research.
Systematic reviewing within the health sciences has almost
always considered evidence arising from 'scientific'
studies. Evidence from randomised controlled trials
(where an intervention is tested against a pre-determined
set of criteria and people are randomly allocated to a
group receiving a given intervention or to a control group)
is usually preferred, as this method attempts to reduce the
possibility of selection bias and other external sources of
bias. Evidence is also considered from other statistical
studies, but they will tend to be considered less important
in an 'hierarchy' of evidence. While critiques can be
levelled at the purity of any 'scientific' study, it is obvious
that many social care interventions are not, by their
nature, amenable to quantitative measurement. The
impact or outcomes of such interventions are often
qualitative rather than quantitative as recipients do not
move to an end 'improved state' in the same way as with
many medical interventions. Interventions are often part

of a complex package of care delivered over long periods of time, thus outcomes are effected by multiple factors and the effectiveness of any one intervention is difficult to evaluate. Establishing control groups can be practically impossible when looking at some social care interventions, as well as raising many ethical questions about depriving one group of people of a service as a means of study. In addition, understanding how service recipients feel about support services and the meaning they ascribe to them (sensitive or soft outcomes) are judged to be as important as hard outcomes in many evaluations of social policies. As a consequence, qualitative methods, alongside or instead of quantitative methods, are used to appraise interventions. However, to date, the techniques of systematic reviewing have given most attention to the quantitative aspects of the review: only recently have social scientists begun to develop new methods of imposing quality criteria on qualitative research (for example, see Popay et al, 1998).

Despite the limitations of the method of systematic reviewing for this area of study, the overall framework within which such reviews are conducted in the health science field was used as the starting point for this study. The main stages involved in undertaking a systematic review are described below. For a full step-by-step process, readers should refer to Deeks et al's (1996) more detailed guide on systematic reviewing.

Defining the scope of the review

The first stage of any systematic review process involves setting the scope and definitional parameters of the review. It is obviously important to account for the area of interest as precisely as possible.

In this study the overall aim of the systematic review was:

> To examine the effectiveness of low intensity support services in enabling people to live independently in their own home.

However, this aim requires further explanation and definition. First, there is no commonly agreed definition of low intensity support services. A working definition of 'low intensity services' was therefore devised for the study:

> Low intensity services are services whose main purpose is to provide general, non-specialist support with daily living skills, practical tasks or emotional support which promotes or maintains a person's ability to live independently in their own home.

Support services were envisaged to be providing assistance with tasks such as:

- moving into a tenancy;
- practical skills such as paying bills and budgeting;
- independent living skills such as cooking, domestic tasks undertaken both inside and outside the home;
- general emotional support;
- befriending and companionship;
- developing social links;
- general advice and information on services and resources within the community.

The support could encompass assistance with tasks which involved the support worker or volunteer directly undertaking that task, or enabling the person to undertake the task themselves. Specialist services provided by trained professionals such as community psychiatric nurses and social workers were excluded, even if they delivered some low intensity support in their role. Home care services were also excluded on the basis that they usually delivered both personal (high level) and practical support (low level).

The aim of the services in helping people 'to live independently' also requires further consideration. The term defies easy definition. The community care legislation sought to enable people "to live as independently as possible" (DoH, 1989) in their own homes or in a 'homely' environment – which effectively included some forms of more institutional provision. In contrast, the term 'independent living' is a recognised concept, developed by the disability movement. Here, independent living, underpinned by a social model of disability, is essentially about equal opportunity and citizenship for disabled people (Kestenbaum, 1996). It emphasises choice and disabled people having access to the support they need, including for many people a high level of personal assistance support. In the field of learning difficulties, however, 'independent living' has not achieved the same influence, and has traditionally been understood as living with no support (Simons, 1997).

For the purposes of this review, services to help people 'live independently' have included only services delivered to people *in their own ordinary housing* (all tenures were included). Services were therefore included irrespective of funding source, whether it be Housing Benefit, Supported Housing Management Grant, social services, joint finances and so on. In this respect, the review looked at support services which were broader than those defined in *Supporting people*.

All forms of institutional or specialist schemes which tied in the provision of housing and support were excluded from the review. Sheltered housing was excluded as it was assessed as specialist provision, even though people had their own tenancies and received low level support. It was also excluded because the effectiveness of sheltered housing arguably deserves its own review. All types of low intensity support services delivered in other settings, for example, day centres and advice centres, were also excluded.

The review included services for any and all groups of people with support needs including the main community care groups (people with learning difficulties, people with mental health problems and older and disabled people) as well as young people, homeless people, those with substance misuse issues, or people experiencing psychological trauma (for example if fleeing domestic violence).

The review was confined to British evidence and to the last 10 years for both reasons of feasibility and applicability to the present day context.

The literature search

Three main stages were involved in the literature search:

- identification of databases and other literature sources to be searched;
- devising a search strategy;
- recovering the literature.

Identification of databases and other literature sources

The NHS Centre for Research and Dissemination (Deeks et al, 1996) identifies a number of areas which need to be considered in a literature search, including:

- electronic databases;
- identification of randomised controlled trials;
- scanning reference lists;
- hand-searching of key journals;
- grey literature;
- conference proceedings;
- consultation with leading researchers and practitioners.

This review utilised all of these methods of literature searching, as well as a website search of leading organisations working in the area.

Appendix A shows the full list of databases searched, along with details of the hand-searches undertaken, Internet searches and contact with key informants. A total of 15 databases (plus a number of allied/sister databases) were searched in the review:

- eight social science databases (for example Social Sciences Citation Index);
- five specialist health databases (for example MEDLINE);
- the Cochrane Library containing databases on randomised controlled trials;
- the British Library grey literature database.

All databases were searched by a trained Information Scientist based in the NHS Centre for Reviews and Dissemination, University of York.

The selection of other sources of information was organised on a less scientific basis. Inevitably hand-searching of library resources was limited by the stocks in the libraries used. The Internet searches and contacts with key informants were pursued through a snowballing method, with links to other websites and one informant recommending another being chief sources of new information. The reason for pursuing these further information sources was to make the review as up-to-date as possible and include research which was perhaps just about to be published, but which would not be included in the databases.

Devising a search strategy

A key part of the process of undertaking systematic reviews involves drawing up a comprehensive search strategy which will, it is hoped, identify all of the relevant literature on a subject. This is a difficult task and, at the end of the day, an imprecise science: one can never know whether the search was correctly targeted but wide enough to capture all the possible research studies in an area.

The full search strategy is outlined in Appendix B. The search terms were, in the first instance, developed and tested on one database (DHData). The search strategy was then tested on a further two databases (the King's Fund and Nuffield databases), and further refined before use on the full range of databases.

The strategy was composed of three sections:

- a first section using keywords and terms to search for different types of services likely to deliver low intensity support services;
- a second section which narrowed the search to include the nature of help or assistance likely to be delivered by such services;
- a stand-alone section of those key areas or services considered to be essential to the search (for example all records on 'floating support' were to be included).

The search strategy also specified that only those records published in or after 1988, and those pertaining to the UK should be included.

Recovering the literature

The databases were searched over a number of months in the autumn of 1999. A total of 5,000 plus references were retrieved. Each reference needed to be checked according to the procedures outlined below: this process was inevitably very labour intensive. A large number of articles and books had to be ordered via inter-library loans or directly in order to assess their suitability for the review.

Although the literature search was comprehensive, a relatively small amount of literature in the subject area was retrieved. As expected, some databases were more useful than others, particularly the databases which included information on reports as well as journal articles. The databases focusing on social care tended to be more helpful than those focusing on healthcare interventions. Searches of key housing and social care newsletters alongside contacting leading organisations or researchers proved valuable in identifying recent and forthcoming reports on low level support.

Selection of studies and data extraction

Following the literature search, the studies to be included in the review had to be selected. This process was assisted by the use of a set of inclusion/exclusion criteria designed to test relevance to the overall study design. For a study to be included, all of the questions required a positive response.

Inclusion/exclusion criteria

1. Is the paper concerned with an examination of a support *service or intervention* designed to help people live independently? (Papers discussing policy and practice issues more generally were excluded.)
2. Is the service primarily available to people in their *own independent accommodation*? (Services in specialist supported housing, residential or institutional care were excluded, as were services in day centres or other community facilities.)
3. Is the service primarily offering *low level* support to people? (Services offering high intensity support or care services were excluded.)
4. Is it a service directly for people with support needs? (Services for carers or staff were outwith the review.)
5. Is the study *evaluative* rather than descriptive? (Papers solely describing a new service were largely excluded – see below.)
6. Was the study undertaken in Britain? (Studies outside of the UK were excluded.)
7. Was the study published in the last 10 years? (Studies before 1988 were excluded.)

The task of selecting studies was not an easy one: it was not always obvious whether a study should be included or not. More specifically, so few studies were found that met all the above criteria – particularly being evaluative in nature – that it was decided to include primarily descriptive studies where they represented the only example of a particular type of service.

Where a study was included in the review, a data extraction or summary form was filled out (as attached at Appendix C). The template was informed by sophisticated evaluative checklists produced by the

Evidence Based Social Care Policy and Practice Research Team at the Universities of Salford and Leeds, and the NHS Centre for Reviews and Dissemination procedures.

Assessing the research evidence

Ultimately the task of the systematic review is to evaluate the quality of the evidence on the subject under study. Traditional systematic reviewing techniques (see Deek et al, 1996) expect literature – predominately quantitative in nature – to be assessed against a number of measures, most particularly:

- the *validity* of the study: appraising the extent to which the conclusions reached can be justified from the data collected, including:
  - *internal* validity: the extent to which the effect is likely to have resulted from the intervention;
  - *external* validity, or *generalisability*: the extent to which the observed effects are likely to hold true for other populations outside the study;
- the *reliability* of the evidence: a measure of the degree to which the same effects are observed when repeated evaluations are undertaken under different conditions, or by different researchers, or in other words, the consistency of the research evidence.

However, the applicability of such measures in assessing qualitative research continues to be debated. While some social scientists might argue that such measures can equally be applied to evaluating qualitative research, leading commentators in this area (eg Popay et al, 1998) propose that, while similarities exist, so do differences, and that these need to be accounted for in undertaking systematic reviews. For the reader to reach a judgement of qualitative material, the information required is similar to that for quantitative material, including a full explanation of the background to the study, objectives, methods and findings and so on (as outlined in Appendix C). However, Popay and colleagues propose that the different nature of qualitative knowledge means that qualitative research must be assessed, first and foremost, according to how the researcher accords, and privileges, *subjective meaning* from the data. For them, the key question is:

> Does the research, as reported, illuminate the subjective meaning, actions and context of those being researched? (Popay et al, 1998)

In appraising qualitative research, factors such as the richness and depth of the data are important, as is the way that the data is contextualised and how meaning is ascribed to the data. Only then can any meaningful appraisal of the validity of the material be attained.

3

Housing/tenancy support: 'enabling' services

Introducing the research findings

The next three chapters provide the main findings of the systematic literature review. This first section explains how low intensity services have been categorised in these chapters. Chapter 1 referred to the difficulties in defining the boundaries between different types of housing management, support and care services. Unsurprisingly when looking at low intensity support services, however tightly defined (see Chapter 2), definitional issues abound in the literature. The presentation of the results of the systematic review reflects the nature of the literature available in this area. However, more crucially, there appeared to be three main types of low level support discussed in the literature. These three types were not necessarily mutually exclusive of one another, rather they summarised the three main purposes of low level support:

Housing/tenancy support: Services which were designed primarily to instruct and 'enable' people with tasks related to moving into and sustaining their own tenancies, which, once (re-)learnt, people would be able to undertake themselves. Tenancy support was seen as a process and was usually regarded as time limited in some respect.

Direct practical support: Services which were designed primarily to provide direct practical assistance for people in their own homes who were unable (and were likely to remain unable) to undertake basic tasks in and outside the home, in other words 'doing' services.

Emotional/social support: Services which were primarily designed to provide companionship, emotional support or extend social networks for people living alone. Such services could be either of a temporary or long-term nature, usually depending on the client group.

It is acknowledged that the above distinctions were in some respect artificial ones (for example tenancy support often also provides emotional support), but they were helpful in thinking about the different functions of services and in explaining some of the successes and deficiencies of services. For example, some people may require long-term emotional support but shorter-term practical tenancy support, but if the latter is seen as the defining form of provision and is withdrawn, tenancies may fail due to the lack of social support given.

All the studies discussed in this and the next two chapters are listed in Appendix D. A total of 41 studies were included in the review: 20 studies which focused on housing/tenancy support services; eight concerned with direct practical support; 13 focusing on schemes primarily delivering social/emotional support.

Housing/tenancy support

Three main types of housing or tenancy support services were discussed in the literature.

Floating support services

Floating support has been variously defined since it was first coined in the early 1990s. Its first and most precise meaning was dictated by the funding source of the support, namely The Housing Corporation Special Needs Management Allowance (now Supported Housing Management Grant). Floating support was defined as consisting of primarily intensive housing management, with occasional general welfare, care and support tasks and advice on bills or debts being delivered (The Housing Corporation, 1995, cited in Morris, 1995). The defining feature of floating support was that it was attached to the individual not the property (although the support had to be delivered to housing association tenancies) enabling it to float off after a period of time. However, the accepted understanding of floating support soon became much broader: it is now used to describe services being delivered in different tenures, using different funding and delivering a wider range of support services (Morris, 1995). It can be floating in three ways: floating from property to property, floating in and out as people need it and varying by intensity over the time of receipt.

Resettlement services

Resettlement services have a very different history to floating support. The term is most closely associated with the former DSS Resettlement Units which were charged with the task of providing services to assist the resettlement of people with 'an unsettled life-style', that is experiencing long-term homelessness. With the closure of these units, however, resettlement took on a much more direct meaning in attempting to literally resettle people into more permanent accommodation (Dant and Deacon, 1989). In addition, resettlement is now closely associated

with resettlement of homeless people – particularly people
sleeping rough – under the Rough Sleepers Initiative (RSI).
From the early 1990s onwards, some local authorities and
housing associations also began to introduce some
resettlement services as a response to high levels of
abandonment and housing management problems. This
trend has continued. The term resettlement has also been
associated with hospital reprovision arrangements for
people with mental health problems and learning
difficulties, although here the focus of resettlement has
almost always been exclusively on specialist residential
and shared provision, and is therefore not included in this
review.

Many points of similarity exist between floating support
and resettlement services. Sometimes the services are
essentially indistinguishable except by name. However,
generally and often (although not always), resettlement
services are front-loaded services, more practically
orientated and shorter in duration. A typical resettlement
service may, for example, provide a lot of assistance with
the moving and settling in process, establishing direct
debits and so on, and perhaps pull out after three to six
months when the person is established in the tenancy.
Floating support may be delivered to people already in
tenancies and usually for a longer time period.

Other types of housing support

This final category is partly a catch-all category for tenancy
services which do not obviously fall into definitions of
floating support or resettlement. The evaluations
identified in the systematic review encompassed a wide
range of services. Some appeared to be more specialist in
focus than the other services, attempting to address certain
behaviour (such as alcohol abuse or offending), or more
specifically addressing health needs. Others offered more

general support that did not label itself floating support or resettlement.

The main studies found by the review in each of these categories are evaluated below.

The effectiveness of floating support services

The last three years has seen a growing number of evaluations of floating support provision being undertaken, some of which are ongoing. Five main evaluation reports have been produced to date. Below the main features of the schemes are introduced, before considering the methods used in the evaluations and most importantly the measures of effectiveness.

Three evaluations have considered the value of a number of different floating support services:

- Douglas et al (1998): a study which examined user views of the value of floating support services for three client groups, people with mental health problems, young people, and people with a physical impairment, in Scotland;
- CVS Consultants (1999): an ongoing evaluation of Housing Association Charitable Trust's Floating Support Programme to examine the extent to which services are meeting individual needs, with the ultimate aim of producing a good practice guide. The first annual report evaluated six projects, including: two schemes for people with mental health problems (in Bournemouth and the Orkneys); a mixed client group scheme but with many people with offending histories (in Stoke-on-Trent); and two schemes for homeless people, one for young homeless (in London and West Yorkshire).

- Goldup (1999): following a feasibility study on floating support (CVS Consultants, 1997), six floating support schemes were set up in North and Mid Hampshire, five of which have been evaluated. The schemes extended across all tenancies and client groups (although people with mental health problems accounted for 35% of all tenants) and were targeted at people who did not qualify for a care package. The purpose of the research was to test the demand for services, different models and the underlying validity of some of assumptions in the models.

Two evaluations focused on one specific scheme:

- Rho Delta (1997): an evaluation focused on a pilot floating support scheme for people with mental health problems in four London boroughs. The evaluation aimed to identify successful elements of the project and identify barriers to success to aid plans for the future. Most people had severe and enduring mental health problems and were eligible for a care management/care programme approach.
- Widdowson (1997): an evaluation of a floating support scheme in Oxford for anyone over the age of 16 in local authority, housing association or private sector housing.

Readers may also like to note that HACT, the Countryside Agency and The Housing Corporation are funding an evaluation of 23 projects in the HACT Rural Supported Housing Programme which includes floating support schemes alongside a range of other supported housing projects. This research, being carried out at the Centre for Housing Policy, University of York, is due to report in 2001.

The above floating support services were broadly delivering the same range of services: a largely generic service to tenants providing personalised and sensitive individual support with practical tasks associated with independent living, emotional support and access to local resources and services as necessary. As can be seen, many schemes were either cross-tenure and/or cross-client group. The vast majority of users, where this was specified, were of white ethnic origin, although there tended to be a balance of genders. Most schemes operated on a ratio of approximately one full-time staff member to 20-30 users, although some had lower ratios when the schemes were in their early stages. The length of support differed by scheme, ranging from nine months to three years (and one with no official time limit).

Most of the studies involved a multi-method approach to undertaking the evaluation. Most collected project monitoring data on referrals and so on, and included both interviews with key players or stakeholders and users. However, the emphasis differed by study. For example, Goldup (1999) was able to provide information on the characteristics of 258 services users, but was only able to obtain 24 completed feedback questionnaires and no interviews with users. In contrast, the Douglas et al (1998) study focused entirely on user satisfaction and included 21 detailed in-depth individual interviews with users and seven focus groups involving 32 people. Generally, however, only a small number of users were interviewed in the studies and monitoring data did not usually collect much information on outcome measures.

Most of the studies also involved a broad evaluation of the nature and effectiveness of the services. To this end, they tended to examine a mixture of process, output and outcome measures, some concentrating on process and output factors more than others. Most authors recognised that their studies were limited in what they could say about outcomes given timescales and research resources. Outcome measures were not always explicitly stated or discussed, making it difficult for the reader to interpret the findings. However, the most common types of outcomes mentioned in the studies were:

- maintenance of tenancies/lack of abandoned tenancies/prevention of homelessness;
- improved quality of life, including increased confidence and self-esteem;
- (occasionally) reducing social isolation/increasing social contacts;
- (very occasionally) health gains.

Some studies also looked at the extent that support plan objectives were achieved and/or user needs met more generally. User's views were the most common method of measuring whether aims had been met, and user satisfaction was often included as an outcome measure in its own right.

A number of studies reported on the extent of tenancy breakdowns, but often inadequate data was presented to be able to make an assessment of the robustness of the information. Rho Delta (1997) found that there were no 'permanent' breakdowns in tenancies, although he pointed out that most tenants had only been in their property for six months or less. One of the projects evaluated by CVS Consultants (1999) achieved a 91% success rate for sustaining tenancies of those referred by probation services over a period of 12 months and 87% after 18 months. However, another project in the same evaluation did appear to experience quite a high number of abandonments (CVS Consultants, 1999).

An overall high level of satisfaction with the services was reported by most studies (although one study noted that this could have been coloured by the adverse previous experiences of users – Douglas et al, 1998). Users often believed that the service had made a difference to their lives. Qualitative information often recorded users talking about increased confidence, self-esteem and generally feeling better about life. However the richness of the qualitative material varied greatly. No quality of life measures were used within the studies.

Floating support appeared very successful in meeting practical needs – most people felt that the help they needed with filling in forms, budgeting and so on was available as and when required, but the success in meeting emotional and wider social needs was more variable. This included both opportunities to talk on a one-to-one basis, to participate in social activities, and help in becoming involved to a greater extent in the life of the community. One researcher commented:

> It would not appear that floating support actually achieves anything in respect of integrating people into the community socially. Nor does it seek to do so, but it may have the perverse effect of depriving them of contact with their community of interest. (Douglas et al, 1998, p 54)

Widdowson (1997) also drew attention to the lack of focus on the ability and potential for members of the local community (rather than community of interest) to assist with making people integrated into community life. He noted that a range of issues needed to be addressed including issues of choice, poverty, isolation and rejection which "goes far beyond the current perceptions of the role of floating support" (p 51).

Very occasionally, studies looked at health gains – particularly the frequency of relapse or hospital stays for people with mental health problems. Two people had hospital stays in the Rho Delta (1997) study, and only one relapse was experienced out of 26 users in the Bournemouth scheme for people with mental health problems (CVS Consultants, 1999).

A number of other factors concerning service delivery were also important in assessing the success of the services in achieving their aims or user outcomes. First, all studies generally reported high demand for services (for example, Goldup, 1999). However, two studies (Douglas et al, 1998; CVS Consultants, 1999) reported that some users were concerned that their floating support was due to float off, and were worried about their future ability to sustain tenancies successfully. While users were with the service, the flexibility and responsiveness of workers were very important (Douglas et al, 1998). The success of the schemes derived from the right sort of help being delivered, but also depended hugely on the approach of the worker and the quality of the relationship with the users: "the attitude of the worker and the tone and quality of their relationship with the user seems to be crucial" (Douglas et al, 1998, p 54). In addition, administrative processes could be important. For example, in the Housing Association Charitable Trust evaluation (CVS Consultants, 1999) support planning appeared to be a key process in ensuring floating support services worked effectively. Rho Delta (1997) pointed out that the decision period before moving in may have been too short and could have led to early transfer requests.

The effectiveness of resettlement services

Most evaluations on the effectiveness of resettlement services have centred on the RSI, which was first introduced in 1990. Over this time, approximately 5,500 homeless people have been housed in about 3,500 permanent units (of these, about 500 were shared flats), as well as substantial amounts of temporary accommodation also being provided. Until 1997, the initiative was exclusively focused on London and most of the research therefore reflects this. However, in 1997 the initiative was extended to 36 areas outside London and also introduced in Scotland (Yanetta et al, 1999). Four reports have been produced by Randall and Brown – the main evaluators of the original RSI (1994a, 1995, 1996, 1999), and a useful study specifically looking at the reasons for tenancy failure was recently carried out (Dane, 1998). Randall and Brown (1994b) also undertook a study for Crisis looking at the success of three resettlement teams. A number of other studies have also been undertaken – usually focusing on the resettlement of specific groups of homeless people including young people (England, 1998) and older people (Crane and Warnes, 1999). It should also be noted that Shelter recently commissioned an evaluation of its new Homeless to Home project which aims to provide support to homeless families.

Most of the resettlement studies are quite explicitly focused on one main outcome measure: whether, and how well, people settle into and maintain their tenancies. Other indicators are usually also discussed; however, these are often ultimately seen as means of maintaining tenancies (for example, increasing social links so that people are less lonely and therefore more likely to settle into their accommodation). The emphasis on maintenance of tenancies is partly a function of the shorter time periods for which the support is offered, as compared to other types of support. RSI arrangements only specify that housing providers usually have to provide help with resettlement for the first six months of a tenancy. The emphasis on outcomes has also increased as subsequent evaluations have been carried out and the full extent of the importance of *effective* resettlement has been realised by the DETR and the housing providers involved in the RSI (Dane, 1998).

The evaluation of the first phase (1990-93) of the RSI (Randall and Brown, 1994a), using a sample survey of 295 resettled people (two thirds of whom were in permanent housing), found 40% of those rehoused in permanent properties stated that they had not received enough help to settle into their new accommodation. By the second phase (1993-96) (Randall and Brown, 1996), only 11% of tenants (of a sample survey of 100 people rehoused) said that they had not received enough support. In addition, a higher proportion (83% to 75%) were satisfied with their accommodation in phase two compared to phase one. This was despite the fact that the second phase targeted more people with longer histories of sleeping rough than in the first phase. Nonetheless, a quarter of tenants were still not settled, particularly younger people, those sharing accommodation and those people who were dissatisfied with the area and perceived themselves to have a lack of social contacts. Over the period October 1994 to September 1995, 294 tenancies were vacated. Half of these moves were planned but half were the result of abandonment or eviction.

Another study undertaken by Randall and Brown in the early 1990s (1994a), looked at the work of three resettlement teams in London – mainly through questionnaire interviews with resettled homeless people.

While users appeared to have a high level of satisfaction with the service, only one fifth received five or more visits, and a number of problems were evident, including a third experiencing rent arrears and some experiencing feelings of isolation.

Following on from RSI studies, the Dane study (1998) focused in more detail on tenancy failure and the main reasons for this. First, Dane looked at the Clearing House database for RSI accommodation to discover the extent of the problem. At 1 September 1997, out of 4,865 tenancies let since 1990:

- 62% were still in existence;
- 13% transferred or moved in a planned way;
- 16% had failed;
- 9% were listed as 'other'.

However, tenancies were more likely to fail in shared (22%) or supported housing (20%), than self-contained (14%) or mainstream (16%). Men were more likely than women to leave their tenancies in an unplanned way (19% and 10%, respectively). White people who were rehoused were more likely to fail than people from ethnic minorities (21% and 10%); interestingly there was little variation between different age groups.

Second, qualitative interviews were undertaken with 50 RSI tenants successfully rehoused (still in a tenancy over one year later) and 22 ex-tenants (who had abandoned the tenancy or been evicted). The study concluded that there were seven main factors that accounted for tenancy failure in self-contained housing:

- social isolation (often because the tenant had accepted a house in location they did not know or in which they had no contacts):

> An acute and pervasive feeling of loneliness was found to be the most common reason why tenants abandoned their Rough Sleeper Initiative accommodation. (Dane, 1998, p24)

- the person was not ready for independent living at the time they were rehoused (either because they had few skills and/or simply did not feel ready);
- poverty (difficult to make a home; made more isolated; hard to budget; no success with work);
- alcohol or drug addition and/or mental health problems;
- lack of available support services; perceived lack of support from resettlement workers (too few visits in the early days, too little contact after six months);
- not being receptive to support (because of pride, fear, lack of trust or lack of interest);
- lack of access to alternative housing options (lack of possibilities to transfer/move).

The reasons for tenancy success were precisely the opposite to the above. A few factors stood out as key – particularly the fact that people wanted to succeed and felt ready to live independently (that is, the motivation to succeed). The role of the resettlement worker was also seen as critical, particularly in the way that they cared and were able to bolster people's confidence and self-respect. Positive strategies for coping with loneliness, as well as poverty, and sometimes drug and alcohol dependancies, were also key.

The implications for resettlement services include better attention to the preparation and pre-tenancy phase, attention to location of property and to social links, and attempts to increase income for people and ensure they have all the furniture and goods needed. Ongoing support also needs to be available to some people. The recent Randall and Brown (1999) evaluation of the RSI echoed many of these factors, also stressing the need for detailed resettlement plans and monitoring of tenancies, and assistance with engaging in employment and training.

Dane (1998) argued that independent accommodation might not have been the most appropriate living arrangement for some people. The Lancefield Street Centre helped 52 older clients resettle a range of accommodation including residential homes, sheltered housing, shared houses with a non-residential support worker and independent accommodation with resettlement support. A study of this operation by Crane and Warnes (1999) found that the longer period of time the person had been homeless, the more difficult they found it to resettle. Conversely, older residents were more likely to settle.

The study of Capital Youth Link (England, 1998) which provided post-resettlement service to 16- and 17-year-olds (non-care leavers), and later 18- to 24-year-olds, focused on the extent to which the service was successful in enabling young people to live independently. Interviews were carried out with almost half of the young people, a majority of whom were young women and from ethnic minority backgrounds. The service was expected to be available to people for 18 months but most users wanted to use it on an open-ended basis. However, there was qualitative evidence that the service was effective in helping young people to maintain tenancies, helping users settle into accommodation and facilitating a growth in confidence and development of day-to-day living skills.

The effectiveness of other types of housing support

There is, perhaps surprisingly, a lack of studies available evaluating housing/tenancy support broadly defined. This may be partly a function of the fact that many housing support services are now described as either floating support or resettlement. It is known that some local authorities and allied agencies undertake internal evaluations of in-house schemes that they have established; however, these are not usually published and would not therefore be identified in a database search. Examples of this which are known to the author include an evaluation of a tenancy support scheme in York (York City Council, 1997) and one in Haringey (Wray, 1996).

One of the few formal research evaluations in this area is by Pleace (1995) who looked at how local housing authorities were responding to the support needs of statutorily homeless single people who were accepted for rehousing. A number of services in operation in four case studies were described but it was also found that the lack of interagency working – most essentially with community care services – worked against the support schemes ability to achieve their aims of ensuring that 'vulnerable' people were adequately supported to maintain their tenancy effectively. In addition, a report was produced by Elsmore in 1996 which analysed the practices of local housing authorities in London in providing support for people with mental health problems. While this report was mainly descriptive it served to highlight good practice in partnership working in this area by local housing departments.

The systematic literature review also discovered a number of studies which, while sometimes termed housing support, were often more specialist in nature. Here, the outcome of maintenance of tenancies was often seen as a means by which to achieve the ultimate objective of improving health and behavioural outcomes. The main outcomes mentioned in the literature were:

- helping people to reduce or manage drug and/or alcohol misuse (Sandham, 1998; Morrish, 1996);
- helping people to address offending patterns (McIvor and Taylor, 1994; Sandham, 1998);
- increasing mental health stability and reducing hospitalisation (Handyside and Heyman, 1990; Warner et al, 1998).

Addressing drug and/or alcohol misuse

The Housing Support Project – part of Coventry and Warwickshire Substance Misuse Initiative – attempted to address both drug abuse and offending patterns by helping support serious drug users with housing problems into stable accommodation (Sandham, 1998). People with substance misuse problems are offered dedicated tenancies conditional on the involvement of a support worker (it should be noted that here the accommodation is, in effect, tied to the support): six month tenancies in the first instance, but permanent tenancies are given after six months if the person has successfully managed the first six months. One of the main aims of the project is to reduce people's drug misuse and thereby reduce crimes committed to sustain their drug habit. From 1995-97, 31 people were offered tenancies, 28 took them up, 13 had completed tenancies, eight were current tenancies and seven had been evicted. The vast majority of clients were male, with an average age of 28. Unfortunately, only four interviews were conducted with users but detailed case records were studied. While there were a number of evictions, some of the successes of the scheme included:

- significant move to use of less serious, and legal, drugs by tenants;
- money spent on drugs declined substantially (from average of £235 to £54 per week);
- associated health gains;
- possible reduction in scale of local drugs market.

However, the evidence on re-offending was not clear (nine of the group had committed new offences) but some people were committing less serious offences than before.

Research undertaken by Shelter (Morrish, 1996) focused on support for problem drinkers through the study of five housing management case studies and 26 interviews with problem drinkers. In addition, a number of descriptive case studies were given of housing support projects for this client group, for example the Alcohol Recovery Project/Phoenix housing management support scheme. While this was not a service evaluation as such, it again shed light on some of the key issues in sustaining tenancies for this group. Interviews with problem drinkers (the majority were men) revealed that one in every three tenancies held had been abandoned. The main reasons for this included loneliness and increased drinking due to social isolation as well as debt. Housing managers associated problem drinkers with violent incidences, vandalism and neighbourhood disputes. The study concluded that standard housing management services were inadequate for supporting these people, with most problem drinkers speaking of the potential value of practical services and companionship.

Helping people to address offending patterns

The Sandman study (1998) above could not prove that the housing support service had had a positive impact on re-offending. The only other study in this area focused on supported accommodation for ex-offenders in Scotland (McIvor and Taylor, 1994) which included an examination of a dispersed model of supported accommodation run by SACRO which aimed to help ex-offenders live more independent lives and prevent further offending. However, while people were offered single-person flats (or in some cases shared flats), they had an occupancy agreement rather than a tenancy, although, as with the Coventry scheme, users could graduate to a permanent tenancy. The project was fairly specialist and involved a structured work programme looking at offending behaviour. It found that very few ex-offenders left the projects in a planned way, most asked to leave or disappeared. While staff were highly regarded, the fact that staff were both providing support and supervision relating to tenants' criminal conviction appeared to negatively affect outcomes.

Stabilising mental health/reducing hospitalisation

Warner et al (1998) brought together findings of five evaluations of services providing support to people with severe mental illness living in their own homes, or what they termed 'extended community support services'. Services provided included practical support within and outside the home, emotional support and help with social activities as well as liaison with statutory agencies and families/carers. A number of outcome measures were used in the studies including sociodemographic data and mental health history; a staff-administered standardised questionnaire designed to measure social and behavioural functioning (Life Skills Profile), both at referral and later; information on inpatient bed use; interviews with users; a quality of life schedule and a standardised rating scale of satisfaction with services. A number of benefits from the services were observed:

- in one scheme there were significant improvements on a number of measures of the Life Skills Profile in the first six months of the service (although no further changes in the next six months);
- a marked reduction in inpatient bed use in another scheme;
- there was a high level of satisfaction with services, and users felt that their social skills and self-confidence had improved (although it did not help them make new friends).

However, one project, while finding high levels of satisfaction, did not find significant changes in social functioning or quality of life over the first six months using the measures, with the exception of subjective questions which asked whether people were feeling better. The authors commented:

> When evaluating support services, some objective measures can be used to assess whether users maintain or improve their social and behavioural functioning, and whether their contact with statutory services decreases. However, the subjective quality of life 'feel-good factor' is an important indicator for services aiming to support isolated people with severe long-term mental health problems. Although there may be no objectively measured improvements in users' quality of life, if they feel better and are more positive about their lives, this is clearly a beneficial outcome. (Warner et al, 1998, pp 41-2)

Another study (Handyside and Heyman, 1990) looked at the impact of a voluntary agency in the North of England which aimed to provide clients with support to reduce the likelihood of hospitalisation. This study looked at the mental health of a small sample of clients (using a Circumstances and Health questionnaire) both before they used the service and after three months of receiving support, and used a control group in two other local authorities. Here they found a statistically significant improvements in mental health for both service users and control groups. However, questions were raised as to whether three months was a long enough period of study and whether the sample was too small.

Finally, while not strictly falling within the scope of the review, it is worth briefly noting studies which have focused on the role of non-professionally trained support workers based in community mental health teams. A Sainsbury Centre study (Murray et al, 1997) asked users in 12 teams (44 users in total) to compare the value and their satisfaction with support they received from a community support worker as compared to their keyworker (usually a trained social worker or community psychiatric nurse). Support workers were seen as significantly more available, more likely to understand user needs and, to a lesser extent, more trustworthy than keyworkers. Emotional support was seen as the most important type of support received from support workers (87% said it was very important), followed by finance (75%), household tasks (58%), medication (53%) and social networks (51%). The study also observed the effect of having support workers in the team on other team members and found evidence that nurses actually adopted a broader role and social workers slightly increased levels of social and emotional support, in teams where support workers were present. While it freed up professionals' time in some cases, it also made them more likely to perform tasks associated with lower-level support. Another survey (Johnson and Brooks, 1997) undertook a national survey of the working methods of community support workers but felt that the effectiveness of community support workers had not yet been conclusively proven.

Conclusion

While a fair number of studies have been undertaken on housing or tenancy support services, most have been small scale in nature, and while occasional studies have collected high quality qualitative information, other studies have conducted very few user interviews and quantitative measures are generally poorly developed. Nonetheless, similar conclusions are drawn by most studies including:

- the way services are delivered obviously has an impact on effectiveness (services need to be flexible, and in some cases long-term);
- services are generally highly regarded by users;
- emotional support/assistance with developing social links is perhaps the most crucial area as perceived by users but often the least well developed.

Subjective measurements of service outcomes are obviously crucial, but it is clear that more objective measures and better monitoring information are required to evaluate other outcomes.

4

Direct practical support

The previous chapter focused on housing and tenancy support services – a major focus of these services is the provision of practical assistance with tasks such as moving in, setting up direct debits for bills and so on. A distinction was drawn that these services are usually undertaken *with* rather than *for* the person, enabling them to become independent and eventually to undertake the tasks in the future with less or no assistance. This chapter focuses on those practical services which are usually carried out *for* the person. Such services may variably provide assistance with tasks such as cleaning, laundry, shopping and collecting prescriptions, assistance with decorating, gardening and household repairs and maintenance. These services tend to be directed at older and disabled people.

The literature on direct practical support services

Virtually no studies evaluating the effectiveness of practical support services were found in the literature search. Given the extent of practical support services such as home help and cleaning services, this is perhaps a little surprising. However, the shift away from these types of services to home care services more generally probably explains the lack of studies: evaluations tend to be undertaken of new initiatives rather than service interventions which are out of favour and being withdrawn. With the exception of one recent Joseph Rowntree Foundation funded report (Clark et al, 1998), the studies that do exist tend to be largely descriptive in nature and are usually one-off, local studies, looking at specific schemes. Due to the dearth of effectiveness studies in this area, descriptive studies have been included where no evaluative studies exist.

Most studies of the value of low intensity direct practical support services focus on services for older people. A further limitation to the research evidence is that it is generally accepted within the research community, that there are difficulties involved in drawing conclusions about user satisfaction from studies of older people given their tendency to not want to criticise services.

The main types of services which have been reviewed in studies over the last 10 years are listed below, and described in more detail in the rest of the chapter:

- housework and domestic services;
- shopping services;
- handyperson schemes;
- good neighbour schemes;
- other miscellaneous services.

Housework and domestic services

A few studies were undertaken at the end of the 1980s/ early 1990s at the time that domiciliary services – particularly home help services – were starting to be reduced. For example, the Cicely Northcote Trust (Lewis, 1988) published an overview of domiciliary services, highlighting good practice and raising issues for discussion. In 1992, the Royal Association for Disability and Rehabilitation (RADAR) and Arthritis Care published a campaigning report highlighting the state of the home help service available for disabled people. However, these studies did not focus on effectiveness and the literature search identified no studies in this area during the mid-1990s, until the Joseph Rowntree Foundation-commissioned report in 1998 (Clark et al, 1998).

The Clark et al (1998) report focused on the value of low level preventative services from the perspective of older people. While this study looked at other areas in addition to housework, including gardening, house repairs and maintenance, laundry and opportunities for social participation, the central emphasis of the study appeared to be domestic assistance as provided, or commissioned, by local authorities, as well as privately-paid home help style services. The study sought to answer three main research questions: What matters about these services? Does it matter who the provider is? Are the services about 'being cared for', or supported in independence? The study took a qualitative approach, undertaking in-depth interviews with 51 older people in their own homes – a third of whom were interviewed more than once to look at changing situations, as well as consultation with a pensioners' group and key stakeholders. The fieldwork was conducted in three local authority areas in Southern England: one city (where most of the interviews were conducted); one rural area; and a conurbation.

A number of Clark et al's (1998) findings are relevant to understanding the importance of, and the key to the effectiveness, of low intensity services. First, the study clearly pointed out how older people made a distinction between 'help' and 'care': the former could be given without undermining their concept of independence as the support was perceived as helping them to look after themselves (in contrast, professionals were much more likely to see older people as 'dependent'). The fact that older people did not have to rely on family (and friends and neighbours) as much for help, enhanced their independence and was seen as a major benefit. In fact, housework was often seen as being as important as care in helping to maintain independence, as one service user commented: "Why is it that home care cannot do any housework because that is important as much as anything else isn't it – to someone who can't do housework?" (Clark et al, 1998, p 21). Help with housework and domestic activities was highly valued by older people. This was particularly the case for older women. Here, being able to keep up the appearance of the home was linked to their sense of identity and feelings of competence – and therefore quality of life. This was particularly important given the many hours that older people spent at home. Simple tasks such as the washing of net curtains were seen as crucial for older women. As the authors, and one older woman, respectively commented:

> The home is not simply a physical environment: it can encapsulate the public and private identity of the older person. Their ability to manage the physical environment and be seen to do so impacts upon their well-being and sense of self as a competent adult member of the community. (p 64)

> "Well you go down if you let your house go down, don't you? If you're not troubled about the house, you're not troubled about yourself, are you?" (p 19)

The study also found that, for many older people, as studies of tenancy support scheme revealed, the relationship with the home help or other worker was as important as the practical help they received. Consistency of staff was therefore key to the benefits gained from the service for older people (again, in contrast providers could sometimes see these relationships as problematic).

While the study did not couch the findings in terms of outcome measures, it was clear that the services provided a number of important outcomes to older people, many of which would have been impossible to measure, but were nonetheless stark, including improved feelings of worth, the retention of a sense of control over one's life and an important emotional/social link with a person whose time and relationship they valued enormously. While it was not possible for the study to categorically state to what extent this might have enabled people to remain living independently, there can be no doubt that it had some impact. The authors concluded that the challenge for policy makers was to look beyond the boundaries of what they perceived as important, and to take on board what older people themselves valued in terms of maintaining their independence.

Shopping services

No specific evaluations of shopping services were found, just two descriptive studies. In 1988, Jervis reported on the Liverpool Shopping Delivery Service which involved young trainees with learning difficulties delivering shopping to older people from a Tesco supermarket. The scheme run by Mencap and Liverpool Social Services was funded from the then EEC Social Fund and Urban Programme as it was providing training. The trainees were employed by Mencap but wore Tesco overalls and shared facilities with Tesco staff. No evaluation was carried out although it was reported that customers were full of praise for the scheme, and the scheme also offered valuable training opportunities to people with learning difficulties.

The second paper described the experience of teleshopping services set up in Gateshead and Bradford (Cahill, 1993). The Gateshead Shopping and Information Service, run by Tesco, the local council and the University of Newcastle, had 1,000 users – mainly older people – in 1988, ordering their shopping at day centres, libraries, residential homes and/or through shopping clerks visiting their home. Of these users, 45% were housebound. However, following the introduction of a charge numbers fell significantly. The Bradford Centrepoint Teleshopping and Information Service, organised by Morrisons had a similar set-up, but was closed down in 1988 by a new council. The paper also reported on a newer service run by Asda. Cahill commented that such services were relatively undeveloped and suggested that the benefits of teleshopping may have included access to cheaper products and not having to rely on others, and could be particularly useful for people in rural areas. Possible disadvantages included taking away the pleasure derived from going out and meeting people when shopping, and the psychological benefits of shopping. While these shopping schemes did appear to prove somewhat unsuccessful with funders, if not with the users, with the advent of the Internet, there is the obvious possibility that increasing numbers of older and/or disabled people and other housebound people can now order their groceries, as well as a range of other products, over the Internet and have them delivered to their door.

Handyperson schemes

Two studies have been undertaken which focus specifically on the value of handyperson schemes for older people (Adam, 1992; Appleton, 1996). In addition, the Clark et al (1998) study included views on these schemes, and Care and Repair England are currently undertaking a study looking at the diversification of Home Improvement Agency (HIA) services. The HIA services include a New Deal handyperson project, hospital discharge scheme and an 'enhancing daily living independence' experimental project, as well as a feasibility study focusing on the provision of gardening being conducted in one HIA.

Older people, especially those over 75, are more likely to live in poor housing, have problems with declining health, have a low income, and possibly also a concern with safety. For this reason, HIAs were set up in late 1970s, with support from the government but coordinated by Care and Repair with the involvement of Anchor Trust, to help older people carry out improvements and repairs on their homes. In 1989, Care and Repair and Anchor Trust raised money from Sainsbury's Monument Trust for three HIAs to directly employ part-time handypersons (for two days a week) to carry out small repairs, adaptations and odd-jobs around the house including essential decorating, putting up curtain rails, repairing electrical appliances and so on. Monitoring over a period of 26 months saw 972 jobs completed for 844 clients. There was a high level of demand for decorating, although this was rationed to essential decorating due to scarce resources and the time-consuming nature of the work. Jobs were only carried out where the work was unlikely to be carried out otherwise (either due to cost or the lack of a contractor). An assessment of client satisfaction undertaken via a postal survey found that the vast majority were very satisfied with the work and, more importantly, over three quarters (78%) said there had been an improvement in their day-to-day living as a result of the work. In 42% of cases the repairs prevented further deterioration of the house.

People appreciated the helpful, friendly staff and the promptness and reliability of the service. The Clark et al (1998) study showed that feeling safe in the home was very important and that, in this context, handyperson schemes were seen as offering a useful service as older people knew that the 'helpers' could be trusted.

A larger survey and evaluation of handyperson schemes was carried out in the mid-1990s (Appleton, 1996). This study identified 63 schemes in England and Wales, three quarters (73%) of which were related to a HIA. The schemes tended to cover the same areas of services as the Adams (1992) study had documented, concentrating on small repairs and minor adaptations. All schemes primarily provided support to low-income homeowners, although half of the schemes also provided some services to tenants. While most of the beneficiaries of the schemes were older people – predominately older women – two thirds also provided services to people with disabilities regardless of age. As with the Adam's study, high levels of satisfaction were found (with the occasional exception of dissatisfaction with long waiting periods), and a range of benefits were reported: 31% felt their home had become more comfortable, 53% said their home was now safer, and 40% reported it was easier to manage. In addition, many users felt more positive about their home and themselves as a result of the work undertaken. The study concluded that handyperson schemes played an important role in enabling older people to remain in their home and brought beneficial effects for health, safety and well-being.

Good neighbour schemes

Three reports were found on the role of good neighbour schemes in supporting people – particularly in rural areas.

However, no studies were retrieved which had been written in the last 10 years and were evaluative in nature. Rather, reports available on good neighbours tended to be essentially descriptive and/or focused on the setting up and management of such schemes.

Clark (1991) undertook a study for the Joseph Rowntree Foundation looking at the practical arrangements involved in setting up good neighbour schemes in villages. He concluded that good neighbour schemes have a key role to play in village life from an examination of six schemes around the country. These schemes undertook activities such as transport, visiting, emergency services (for example, following bereavement), advice, information and counselling (although this was mainly left to organisations such as Citizens' Advice Bureaux), collecting prescriptions, disability aids, and arranging day centres and call-in clubs. The study stressed the need for fixing boundaries to the service, identifying needs, having a committee and a coordinator for each scheme, and having procedures for the recruitment, training and support of volunteers. Clark (1991) asserted that such schemes could bring communities closer together, as well as stimulate other activities.

A study of the contribution of good neighbour groups to community care in the county of Gloucestershire was undertaken by Short (1993). The study identified 25 groups in the area and surveyed them to provide details on their operation. Case studies of eight of these organisations looked at the organisational arrangements of the schemes through interviews with coordinators, including their relationships with statutory organisations and recruitment and deployment of volunteers. As with the other studies, no data were available on the value of the service from users' points of view. Short (1993) recommended the need for a centralised body to support the development of groups in the county.

McCullagh and Rich (1996) reported on a Church of England-led initiative in Hampshire to set up a network of neighbourhood groups, where volunteers were helping to improve the quality of life of housebound people by taking them to the hairdresser and doing simple practical tasks such as changing light bulbs and so on. Here, the importance of paid advisors and a steering group was stressed to ensure the effective delivery of services.

Miscellaneous services

An interesting study was undertaken by Franklin (1996) into the role of concierges in tower blocks in Glasgow. While the role of concierges falls broadly within the housing management service of the council, this study illustrated that these caretakers had developed their social and welfare role to offer a variety of services to tenants, many of which were essentially low level, direct practical support services.

As a response to housing management problems in the area, 24-hour concierges were introduced into 91 tower blocks in Glasgow in the early 1990s in an attempt to increase security as well as to strengthen the relationship between the housing service and tenants. While paying due care and attention to the security and cleaning aspects of their job, helping tenants who often had support needs was seen by concierges as a major part of their role. The authors noted that:

> [Concierges] take a real pride in their willingness to assist tenants with anything they are asked to do [including] administration of first aid; changing

light bulbs; cleaning windows; assembling
furniture; minor electrical repairs; moving heavy
objects; carrying shopping; 'doing the carrots';
hanging curtains; looking after people's keys
during the day; making early morning calls;
making cups of tea for people using the laundry;
fetching prescriptions; contacting home helps;
fund raising for pensioners outings. (Franklin,
1996, p 33)

It was also noted that concierges spent a great deal of time
chatting to people and were willing to be called upon by
lonely individuals who simply wanted someone to talk to,
and, as they worked 24 hours a day, to console or comfort
people at any time of day or night. The authors made
comparison between the role of concierges and warden
services; their role might also be compared to a hostel
reception worker. While tenants in the tower blocks were
not interviewed it was suggested that this service might be
valuable to people with support needs such as older
people and people with mental health problems or
physical impairments.

As stated at the outset, sheltered housing services fell
outside the remit of this project. However, it should be
noted that peripatetic wardens now exist who deliver low
level support (for example, pop-in calls) to people who
live in the their own homes in the local community as
well as sheltered housing tenants. While no specific
evaluations of these schemes were found, their potential
role is clear. The role of such wardens also ties in with
the more specific role of now widespread community
alarm systems. A number of studies exist on the value of
community alarms. These are not considered in this
study, as services delivering mainly a monitoring role,
rather than a support one, were excluded from the review.

However, studies such as Thornton (1992) have highlighted how the technology cannot stand alone – for such a service to be effective the alarms should act as a personal support service, as there is often a need for a listening ear and/or practical help in small matters as well as an emergency service.

Conclusion

The systematic review process uncovered very few high-quality research studies on the effectiveness of low intensity direct practical services. This is likely to reflect the low emphasis placed on them in policy, and the lack of evidence is also likely to do little to assist their future development, even though the little evidence that does exist suggests that people place a high value on such services. However, outcome measures to capture the benefits of such schemes, for example, looking at the extent to which direct practical services improve quality of life and can help prevent older people moving into residential care, are yet to be designed.

5

Emotional and social support

Over one quarter of the population now lives alone, and while loneliness may be a problem for anyone within this group, it is likely to be much worse for people with support needs. A majority of people with support needs are unable to work, either due to health problems, age and/or due to lack of opportunities available to them in the labour market: opportunities for socialising at work are therefore not possible. In addition, it has been shown that people with support needs generally have smaller networks of friends and social contacts, this is particularly true for people with mental health problems where it has been shown that when people become ill, friendship networks dwindle significantly (Hamilton et al, 1989, cited in Bradshaw and Haddock, 1998). Further, there is a substantial body of research which demonstrates the impact that loneliness and a lack of social support can have on both physical and psychological health status (see Andersson, 1998; Uchino et al, 1999) and for older people, the risk of moving to residential care and of mortality (Bowling, 1991). The importance of ensuring that people's emotional and social needs are met therefore cannot be underestimated.

As the two previous chapters showed, the relationship between a support worker, whether that be a tenancy support worker or home help, and a user, is highly valued by users. While some services already described, such as floating support, attempted to provide emotional support as well as practical support, this was often a minor rather than a major aim and they were often found to be lacking in this area. This chapter focuses on the effectiveness of services which had the prime (if not only) aim of providing emotional and/or social support to people with support needs living independently in their own homes.

The main types of services identified in this area were:

- mutual support networks;
- friendship schemes;
- befriending services;
- homevisiting services;
- telephone support services;
- virtual social support;
- other services.

These services worked on a number of different levels. In the case of most services, the relationship between the volunteer or worker and the user was seen as central to addressing emotional needs. In the case of services such as homevisiting, it was the main focus. Other services such as mutual support networks also aimed to help people form social links beyond the relationship between the helper and the service user, here, in the form of providing links with other people in their community of interest (that is, other people with similar support needs) through developing group networks. Other schemes, particularly befriending schemes, also attempted to help people make social links within the wider community. The main aim of these services was to reduce loneliness and increase social links and participation in the community. Often these aims were couched in terms of the 'integration' of people into communities; however, a number of other outcomes were sometimes mentioned, including reducing health problems (for example, depression), reducing the risk of relapse (for example, for people with addictions) and reducing the risk of moving to residential care (particularly for older people). Here, a reduction in social isolation was seen as a means of, as well as an end to, preventing health deterioration, reflecting the concerns in the literature mentioned earlier.

The services reviewed provided emotional and social support to all user groups, although each individual scheme tended to be provided specifically for one group of people with support needs. The services were also provided for varying lengths of time, but in general, the intention of most of the support was that it would be ongoing unless the user decided otherwise. This was often made possible by the fact that many social support schemes utilised the service of volunteer visitors or befrienders, meaning that the issue of funding was a less pressing one than where paid workers were involved (although still not absent). The previous chapter showed that volunteers were sometimes used to deliver low intensity practical support, particularly in good neighbour schemes. Such schemes often also offered visiting as a service in itself. It is with social support schemes that the use of voluntary assistance really takes centre stage in the provision of low intensity services.

Below, the evidence on the effectiveness of the main types of services listed above are reviewed.

Mutual support networks

Two evaluations of what have been termed 'living support networks' have been undertaken. Simons (1998) undertook an evaluation of KeyRing – a low level support service which was set up in the early 1990s to provide long-term housing and support for people with learning difficulties. In 1995, the Home-Link scheme was established, based on the KeyRing scheme, to provide a similar service for people with mental health problems and evaluated by Quilgars (1998). Both evaluations used in-depth interviews with users as the main method of evaluating the success of the projects, as well as carrying out additional interviews with staff, volunteers and key players, and an examination of costs and organisational structures.

The main principles of both schemes involved housing up to 10 people within walking distance of each other in mainstream tenancies, and offering the support of a part-time community living worker to provide assistance with day-to-day living and the development of a mutual support network between tenants. Both services successfully provided practical, flexible and ongoing support to users, bringing benefits of improved confidence, quality of life and health benefits for both people with learning difficulties and people with mental health problems. The continuous nature of the support was stressed by both schemes: it was acknowledged that people with learning difficulties needed ongoing support and that to withdraw support from people with enduring mental health problems was to risk a person deteriorating and re-entering the psychiatric system at a later date. However, there were some differences between the two schemes (see Quilgars, 1998, and Simons, 1998). For example, in KeyRing, workers were expected to live in a council tenancy in the same area (and received free rent in return for giving 10 hours of support a week) whereas the Home-Link workers were based in agency settings and did not disclose their home address to the users of the scheme.

In addition, one of the major differences between the schemes was their understanding and emphasis on the development of mutual or social links between group members. KeyRing firmly believed in encouraging users to provide support to one another, by requiring them to attend tenant meetings which were held in each other's flats. Home-Link saw this as too invasive for people and preferred to stress the development of social links which were encouraged through voluntary participation in social gatherings held in neutral places. Overall, the KeyRing scheme placed a greater emphasis on community development work than was the case with Home-Link, which probably accounted for their overall greater success with developing mutual support networks compared to Home-Link. While this element of the Home-Link scheme was welcomed and appreciated by users, it was found that few users met with each other outside of the group meetings. There were more examples of mutual support between KeyRing tenants (people doing each other's shopping, re-lighting boilers for others, explaining details about services), although interestingly it was an aspect of the service which tenants underplayed. In both schemes, there were a minority of users who did not wish to participate in this element of the scheme (called 'ghost' tenants in the KeyRing services), which perhaps stresses the importance of providing such a scheme to people who are initially interested in the idea of mutual support.

Friendship schemes

A number of studies have been undertaken which have focused on services which attempt to help people to increase their friendship circles. These services are perhaps best known in the learning difficulties field; however, they almost always focus on the social needs of people living in a range of different housing and support situations. In short, they do not tend to centre their attention on supporting people living independently. This, no doubt, reflects the fact that supported living for people with learning difficulties still remains poorly developed (Simons, 1997). Strictly speaking such services fall outside of the review. For interested readers, examples of studies in this area included Bayley (1997) who worked to increase the friendship networks of people with learning difficulties living in families and hostels as well as independently (interestingly he found that those people in couples seemed more stable than those who were single, highlighting the importance of relationships), and Schneider (1992) which focused on a friendship service centring on the move from hospital to community provision.

Befriending services

In their recent national study of befriending schemes, Dean and Goodlad defined 'befriending' as:

> ... a relationship between two or more individuals which is initiated, supported and monitored by an agency that has defined one or more parties as likely to benefit. Ideally the relationship is non-judgemental, mutual and purposeful, and there is a commitment over time. (1998)

This definition, derived from the Scottish Befriending Development Forum, identifies the fact that befriending is a formal service to the extent that an agency is responsible for selecting and supporting befrienders and for putting these befrienders in touch with interested users. This, in essence, distinguishes it from 'friendship' which has been defined, again by the Scottish Befriending Development Forum, as 'a private, mutual relationship', although it was clear from the studies that on some occasions friendships did develop from a befriending relationship.

Dean and Goodlad (1998), with funding from the Joseph Rowntree Foundation, identified befriending schemes in Britain through the Scottish Forum and contact with half of the social services departments in England. A postal survey to the schemes identified, gave information on 234 schemes (a 70% response rate) and provided a picture of the activities of befriending services. Six case study schemes targeted at different client groups allowed a more in-depth analysis of services and their impact; 28 users (or carers) and 31 volunteers were interviewed in the six schemes. A number of issues arose with 'inputs', as 62% of all schemes stated that it was a problem for them to find volunteers to run the schemes; with 19% also saying they had a problem with recruiting users. Once volunteers were recruited, befriending relationships lasted an average of 12 months in the case studies, with services generally being of shorter duration for young adults, people with mental health problems and other groups compared to older people.

From the user interviews, a number of aspects of the befriending relationship were valued:

- companionship;
- the ongoing nature of contact;
- appreciation of different leisure opportunities (outings etc, although here it was often the possibility of such outings as they often did not happen as much as would have been liked);
- appreciation of the organisation (particularly contact with the coordinator and other staff). (Dean and Goodlad, 1998)

There was, however, limited evidence of broader social

inclusion, although there were some notable success stories. It was also found that users did not value this wider social inclusion as much as the organisations:

> ... this tension is symptomatic of a difference of view about how far users should aspire to the sorts of social network which characterise the lives of volunteers and project co-ordinators. (Dean and Goodlad, 1998, p 45)

In general, the authors pointed out that it was almost impossible to assess the overall effectiveness of such schemes:

> Case study befriending schemes are convinced of the value of what they do, but are unable to demonstrate it with reference to the sort of formal performance measurement methods which have become characteristic features of the way welfare agencies deliver services.... No one could be sure that befriending had made any difference in the users' community participation. If it has increased, it may have done so anyway. If not, the exclusion might have been worse without the befriending....

> Evaluation would have to be more wide-ranging and sophisticated than the adoption of a single target (which would have the danger of subverting some of the purposes of befriending), and would need to take account of the inherent ambiguities of purpose and the intangible nature of befriending's achievements. This issue requires more detailed consideration than it has had here or in most befriending agencies. There is a need for more research. (Dean and Goodlad, 1998, pp 34 and 46)

Notwithstanding this, the literature review uncovered four studies which have attempted to evaluate befriending schemes (Bradshaw and Haddock, 1998; Copello et al, 1998; Harris et al, 1999a, 1999b; Oakley et al, 1998).

The Harris et al (1999a) study represents one of only two randomised controlled trials (RCT) included in the review. The aim of the study was to evaluate a volunteer befriending scheme as an intervention among women with chronic depression in inner-London. The RCT hypothesis was that those allocated befriending would often show more improvement or recovery from depression than a control group (taking account of severity of depression, co-morbidity, duration of illness and other treatment experience). The Islington branch of the Family Welfare Association extended an existing service for the purposes of the research. Befriending was defined as meeting and talking for a minimum of one hour per week, acting as a 'friend' and 'being there' for the person. Women were identified through a postal survey of a number of GP practices (using a version of the General Health Questionnaire) (N=4,182), followed by telephone screening (606) and home psychiatric assessment (104) of those with chronic depression and who were interested in being involved. Forty-three woman were randomly allocated to a control group (who did not receive the service until 12 months later) and 43 to the befriending service. The study found that:

> 65% of those allocated befriending experienced remission from depression (for at least two months in duration) compared to 39% of the control group.

This represented an increase in the remission rate of 43%, which the authors commented was a level of success comparable to those emerging from pharmacological trials for non-chronic conditions.

Harris et al (1999b) subsequently carried out further analysis to examine the potential role of other psychosocial factors which might be relevant to the outcomes of the service, also comparing their study to two further population samples (not receiving a befriending service). They found that 79% of women who experienced 'fresh-start' experiences (for example, meeting a new partner) during the 12 months had remission compared to only 31% of those without. Good coping strategies/attachment style identified at entry to the service also enhanced remission chances, while new adverse life events and poor coping strategies prevented it. However, it was found that befriending still played a role in increasing the chance of remission, over and above the other factors. The logistic regression odds ratios were 4.12 for standard attachment, 6.92 for a fresh-start, 4.51 for absence of new stressor and 4.09 for befriending. This follow-on study revealed that befriending played the greatest role for those not experiencing a fresh-start experience and with either experience of new adverse events or interpersonal difficulties at interview (non-standard attachment). Those in the control group with a fresh-start experience did as well as those allocated befriending.

The Copello et al (1998) study focused on the use of volunteers as befrienders within a community alcohol team. The service sought to provide ongoing support, especially to those isolated in the community, aiming to:

- enhance clients' social networks;
- develop greater community involvement;
- reduce the risk of relapse.

The underlying model for the service was the Community Reinforcement Approach which stresses the importance of social systems that do not support drinking in enabling people to control their drinking. Six volunteers were trained, and 12 clients (eight women and four men, mixed age, most lived alone) were introduced to befrienders, although three did not engage with the service. Befrienders, clients and keyworkers were all given feedback questionnaires asking them about the benefits of the scheme (five clients returned the questionnaire). The main findings were:

- All parties agreed the befriender was supportive; however, progress in enhancement of social networks was not so clear: keyworkers and befrienders thought this had happened in more cases than users.
- While there were only a few relapses in drinking it was difficult to say whether this was due to befriending although befrienders and keyworkers felt contact had helped people manage drinking (again users were less sure).
- It was not very clear whether the scheme resulted in increased involvement of the local community: on some occasions befrienders introduced people to college, local clubs and so on, but a lot of activities were potentially solitary ones, for example, swimming.

The authors were interested in the fact that the clients who did not engage in the service were all male and felt that further investigation was required to discover whether women respond better to this type of service.

The Bradshaw and Haddock study (1998) looked at the value of trained befrienders to people suffering from long-term mental health problems. Again this was a small-scale project, this time examining a befriending service set up

by Making Space and Wigan Health Authority/Social
Services which aimed to enhance users' quality of life by
minimising isolation. Interviews were undertaken with
nine users (five lived alone, four with parents; average age
39; mixed gender). The length of involvement with the
befriender ranged from one to nine months, and contact
ranged from daily to monthly. Those living alone tended
to see the befriender in their own home and activities
centred around this, while for those living with parents,
activities more usually involved getting out of the house.
All service users felt the befriending had been helpful, in
particular:

- no one reported a decrease in social activity,
  confidence or energy and interest in going out;
- 67% of users thought it had improved their self-
  confidence;
- 44% thought that their social activity had increased
  (although four fifths of those living alone reported no
  change);
- 56% felt their opportunities for going out had
  improved.

The main limitation of the Copello et al (1998) study was
the small number of subjects involved, and the short
period of the evaluation.

Finally, Oakley et al (1998) looked at the operation of four
Home-Start schemes primarily aimed at mothers who were
socially isolated and suffering from low emotional well-
being. Such services are essentially aimed at supporting
parenting, rather than independent living per se, but the
study was included due to its relevance to befriending
services to people isolated in the community. While the
authors noted that the research was essentially descriptive,
some information was collected on outcomes which

indicated that further investigation may discover that such a service could increase confidence and coping strategies.

When assessing the evidence of the effectiveness of befriending schemes, it is important to note that evidence from a number of studies (for example Dean and Goodlad, 1998; Harris et al, 1999a; Oakley et al, 1998) suggests that a significant proportion of those eligible for, or offered befriending, do not want to participate in this type of service. Such services may therefore only be effective for some people with support needs.

Homevisiting

Homevisiting is looked at separately to befriending as such services usually primarily involve visiting people in their own homes (although some practical assistance and outings may also be arranged), rather than the broader role of befriending in helping people to extend their social links. The main study undertaken on homevisiting was by Salvage (1998) for Age Concern and concentrates on services for older people. The aim of the study was to provide accurate and up-to-date information on the nature of visiting schemes; the study was therefore more descriptive than evaluative. Twenty homevisiting schemes were chosen (to achieve a geographical spread) for study from the Age Concern England Service Database and telephone interviews were undertaken with scheme organisers. Most of the users were women in their 80s and 90s, who were mainly living alone. The author commented that it was not easy to judge the success of the schemes, particularly as 'inputs' and 'outputs' were difficult to define and measure. However, they found a low turnover of volunteers (although there were problems in recruiting volunteers) and that, in many cases, real friendships were established (sometimes people were adopted as a 'granny'). Three of the 20 organisers felt that the schemes prevented a person having to go into residential care, six felt it delayed this, with four commenting that it helped in conjunction with other services. The main achievements, as described by organisers, were: relieving of loneliness and isolation; feeling valued; prevention of residential care; improved quality of life; having something to look forward to; and giving a point of contact with the outside world.

A number of local small-scale evaluations have also been undertaken on homevisiting, for example one was undertaken by Lee (1994) on the Drumchapel Elderly Homevisiting Scheme. While local evaluations can be invaluable in informing the development and future direction of such projects, they are often limited by few resources and may be undertaken by project staff.

Telephone befriending

Age Concern (Scotland) and Engage (Scotland) recently published a report on volunteering from home, looking at the potential for telephone befriending schemes to meet the needs of housebound people to volunteer and of those who would like to be a recipient of the scheme (Age Concern [Scotland]/Engage [Scotland], 1999). The report is part of a three-year Scottish Homes initiative to explore later life volunteering. The research included a comparative study of four telephone study schemes: Gordon Volunteer Centre and Edinburgh and Leith Age Concern befriending service, WRVS West Fife Good Neighbour scheme and Wing Hong Chinese Centre in Glasgow. The study pointed out the value of volunteering by people who may be disabled and have limited mobility, and that little attention has been paid to developing telephone volunteering services. The report also gave the main results of four pilot schemes of telephone befriending for six months (as above except for the Gordon Volunteer Centre) which showed positive feedback from both volunteers and users, with benefits listed as including enhancing quality of life of both users and volunteers, as well as how telephone contact can increase people's participation and awareness of community issues. The report concluded that more demonstration models were required to fully evaluate the schemes.

Virtual social support

Studies are just beginning to be undertaken focusing on the potential of virtual social support – that is, support over the Internet – to meet the support needs of people living in the community. Internet support is potentially useful for those who are housebound, find it difficult to go out or arrange transport, with obvious possibilities in rural areas. Such support is also available on a 24-hour basis and widens the choice of possible relationships beyond the locality and gives the possibility of anonymity. Finally, and most importantly, it is quite different from many other forms of services as it is user-led and tends to be organised and regulated by people with support needs themselves. The possible disadvantages are that it does not involve face-to-face contact between people, which raises questions of how meaningful and useful such distant relationships can be to people (although some people do end up meeting up and/or forming personal relationships outside of the groups). In addition, the technology required to participate in such support is usually only available to groups with adequate income and resources which at present would exclude many people with support needs. Some commentators have also suggested that Internet use may decrease social interaction in other areas (see Pleace et al, forthcoming, for a fuller description of the pros and cons of such provision).

The ESRC has recently funded a project to investigate virtual community care in meeting the support needs of people with different health and support needs, including people with alcohol problems, those suffering from depression and disabled people. One paper produced by the research team at the Universities of York, Teeside and Durham (Pleace et al, forthcoming) examined the use of the Internet relay chat 'room' (allowing synchronous communication) by a group of people recovering from alcohol dependency. It should be noted that these groups tend to attract international users – a feature of the form of provision – so the support will also have been received by a wider, international, audience. The research, which involved anonymous visits (54 in total) by the researcher to the site over five months, found evidence that supportive relationships were present. The researchers found that users gave and received emotional support and reassurance, advice on other resources (as well as referring people on to professional and established services, recognising perhaps the limitations of the service), as well as participating in more general social chat. The main limitation of the research involved the fact that the team were unable to ask users directly whether they found the chatroom helpful.

A second paper by the same team of researchers (Muncer et al, 2000) examined a Usenet newsgroup for people suffering from depression. They looked at a random sample of postings to the newsgroup – 491 messages posted by 118 participants – and found that the majority of exchanges were supportive. This support tended to deliver three types of social support: social companionship, informational support and esteem support (three of the four types of social support in the typology by Cohen and Willis, 1985). There was very little of what has been termed 'instrumental' support (that is, practical support), but this was not surprising given the distance between users. Once again, it was not possible for the researchers to say precisely how useful this support was, but they concluded that the number of posts and the nature of the responses to them suggested significant value. In some cases, examples of social support were quite striking. One user who was, as s/he described it, "crashing big time" replied to other users who had offered messages of support as follows:

> "Hi, me again. After I posted last night I logged off and went to bed. I was delighted to see some caring e-mail in my box this morning.... Thanks it means a lot to me. I'm feeling a little better this morning, at least I don't feel like cutting or drinking or hurting myself. Your support helped a lot ... I love you all so much. Although you don't know me well, I feel like I know you from reading your posts. I feel safe here. Thanks and love to you all."

It is still too soon to evaluate the impact of such a new area of social support. Research methods also need to be developed which will allow better evaluations to be undertaken so that users are consulted and involved in the research. However, the first evidence suggests that virtual social support could offer some people with support needs a number of benefits.

Other services

Two other studies were found which, at least in large part, involved the provision of social and emotional support to people living independently, in this case, older people.

Clarke et al (1992) undertook an RCT involving 523 older people in Leicestershire identified from a GP register in Melton Mowbray, Leicestershire. The older people were interviewed and randomised into an experimental and control group. The control group was offered support from a lay worker to help arrange varying types of support aimed at enhancing people's social contacts, tailored to the user's requests. A number of measures were used to assess the older people's level of cognitive functioning, loneliness, daily living activities and self-perceived status, at the start of the study and 15 months to two years later. The study found no significant differences between the experimental and control group in levels of mortality, physical health, demand for services, nor on some subjective measures such as loneliness. However, the experimental group showed significantly improved self-perceived health status. It was also noted that the measures used to assess social changes judged improvements on the number of social contacts and did not take account of the quality of the relationship between the worker and the user: therefore, the measures may not have been sensitive enough to identify changes in well-being. The study also noted the high numbers of older people who declined assistance.

Finally, a small-scale evaluation was undertaken by Thornton (1995) on the first 18 months' (pilot) progress of the newly established Homeshare Project. The project, based on an idea from Canada and the US, involves a householder – usually an older person – exchanging rent-free accommodation for up to 10 hours of low level support being delivered by the lodger. The support can be of any type including practical assistance and sometimes even some personal care. However, one of the main aims of the service is to offer companionship, as well as the benefits of having someone in the house for reasons of security and so on. Twenty interviews were undertaken with staff/volunteers and householders. While, in the pilot study, outcomes could not be looked at in detail, some potential benefits were identified including increased feelings of safety and increased social well-being (sometimes a new friend; bringing the outside world to older people). The study also suggested that the scheme often worked to the mutual benefit of both parties where companionship was the main reason for the homesharing, but pointed out that it was difficult to contract for the development of such a relationship.

Conclusion

A number of evaluations have been conducted on the effectiveness of social and emotional support, especially befriending schemes. It is clear that such schemes may be suitable for some people with support needs, but may suffer from poor take-up among others with support needs. A number of outcomes appeared likely – particularly around improved confidence and reduction in social isolation through the benefits of a valued relationship and, in one study, stability of health. However, the studies do not appear to indicate that such schemes are especially, if at all, successful in widening people's social networks and fostering 'integration' into the 'community'. Further robust evaluations are required in this area to explore these issues in greater depth.

6

Towards effective services

This final chapter begins by presenting an assessment of the overall value and robustness of the research evidence on low intensity support services. Despite the limitations associated with the evidence base, the chapter outlines what is known about the effectiveness of low intensity services. Finally, the chapter ends by considering what needs to be done to move towards a better evidence base in this area.

Effective evaluations?

While the robustness of the methods used within the studies included in the review inevitably differed from study to study, and some types of services had benefited from more research attention (such as resettlement and befriending) than others (such as direct practical support), overall the body of research evidence on effectiveness in this area was found to be poorly developed. In assessing the validity and reliability of the research evidence and, in the case of qualitative material, how well the research illuminated the subjective meaning of people's situations (see Chapter 2), a number of limitations with the evidence base were evident.

Poorly developed outcome measures

Much of the research in the area of low intensity services is largely descriptive rather than evaluative. Most studies concentrate on inputs and processes, such as referrals, staffing and organisational structure; outcome measures are rarely mentioned explicitly. While studies usually indicate the possible benefits arising from such service interventions, sometimes with good examples, they are rarely able to back this up with robust evidence. The validity of the conclusions of the studies are therefore problematic.

Problems of generalisability

Most studies in the area of low intensity support services have been small in scale, localised to particular areas of the country, and examining services for a small number of users and/or only one user group. Large data sets (with the possible exception of the RSI database) do not appear to exist in this area. This makes the generalisation of findings to other groups of people, in different settings and locations problematic. Even in qualitative research, the small size of samples and a lack of purposive sampling makes generalisability in a theoretical sense difficult.

Measurement over time

Most studies represent snapshots of the success of schemes. Few long-term evaluations have been undertaken which allow outcomes to be measured over time. For example, many studies focus on the stability of tenancies over a 6- to 12-month period, whereas the crucial period of time for succeeding in a tenancy may be longer than this. While a few studies have followed a small cohort of people over time, no longitudinal studies have been undertaken in this area. Linked to this, while studies often collect basic information on user characteristics, more sophisticated use of baseline data is rare, which makes it much more difficult to measure the effects of services over time.

Lack of control of other factors

Very few studies have tried to answer the question: what would have happened if people had not received support from the service?: only two RCTs were found in the review. The use of control groups in evaluating social interventions is fraught with problems. Perhaps the largest problem relates to the fact that social interventions such as low intensity support schemes are often small scale; whereas RCTs need to use samples large enough to enable randomisation to reduce the likelihood of bias in the data. There are also ethical considerations involved in delivering services to some people but not others with similar levels of need. However, these problems may not be insurmountable and require more detailed discussion. On a simple level, the importance of taking account of factors other than the specified service intervention are crucial, for example, one service may appear more effective than another, but if the former intervention is delivered as part of a package of services, and the latter in isolation, the real difference in effectiveness may be smaller than observed.

Assessing subjective accounts

A small number of good quality pieces of qualitative work do exist providing essential insights into people's feelings, experiences and views on service interventions. In these studies, attention is given to the way in which people ascribe meaning to the support and it is possible to begin to understand the difference services may make, and the reasons for these differences (for example, how the meaning of 'home' and gender helps understand the importance ascribed to domestic services by older women; Clark et al, 1998). However, these studies represent the exception to the rule – it is clear that there is still much scope for developing and exploiting the value of qualitative interviewing in future evaluations. However robust statistical monitoring of outcomes becomes, qualitative data will also be required to understand in detail the effects of a service (for example, why tenancies fail or succeed).

Ideological position

Looking at the research studies on low intensity services, researchers rarely make their ideological or value beliefs explicit. While this area of study is not overtly politicised (for example, research is hardly ever written up within a Marxist, radical feminist or similar framework), the implicit ideological approach of the researcher is still likely to impact on the way that the research is carried out and how the findings are interpreted. Within the present body of work, the ideological starting point for many researchers appears to be one that essentially assumes that low intensity support services are a 'good thing'. In many ways this reflects little more than the desire of a social researcher to support social policy interventions designed to improve the lives of people with support needs; however, it may be conjectured (and it is only a conjecture) that this may lead to presentation of findings that would be different to those presented by someone who felt that such services were inherently problematic. It may be that a more explicit discussion of the value base of research studies would be valuable and, may, ultimately lead to more challenging and robust pieces of research being undertaken.

Effective services?

It is clear that the evidence on the effectiveness of low intensity support services, as a body of research, has a number of limitations. This does not, however, mean nothing can be said about the value of low intensity support services; rather it means that areas for further research can be identified. This section considers what can be concluded from a review of research in this area; in short, what services are effective in helping people to live independently successfully?

The first important point to make is that there was no evidence that low intensity support services, of any type, were harmful to people with support needs, or lessened the likelihood of them being able to live independently. This differs to some health or medical interventions which can actually be harmful to a person. It may, of course, be that some problems with the services were not reported in the research studies (perhaps reflecting the value base of the studies) or that the research studies did not ask the right questions to discover the problems with such services. The only problems that did sometimes exist were that services had a low up-take (and may therefore not have been seen as useful by some users), or where services were insufficiently intensive to give a person all the support they felt they needed to live independently. A striking finding was the way that users consistently valued the support of a support worker or volunteer, often in preference to other more formal service interventions (see Murray et al, 1997).

The evidence available on the effectiveness of some types of services was greater than for other services. With this understanding, the key learning points or conclusions from the studies are reviewed below. Five main types of outcomes are considered:

1. Housing outcomes (for example, tenancy stability, lack of rent arrears).
2. User-centred outcomes (for example, feelings of greater control over life, increased self-esteem).
3. Social outcomes (for example, reduced isolation, greater social participation).
4. Health-related outcomes (for example, improved health).
5. Wider community outcomes (for example, reduced crime).

Housing outcomes

While the literature documented some positive housing outcomes, there was a lack of good quality data in this area from which to draw firm conclusions about the benefits of services.

- It is not possible to state the extent to which tenancy/ housing services prevent tenancy breakdown as different services experienced varying levels of success in this area. However qualitative data highlighted the factors which led to tenancy breakdown, indicating that a complex range of factors (including sufficient support, location of accommodation, social networks, motivation of the person, not rushing the decision or the move and so on) did influence tenancy success.
- Some studies indicated that users were concerned that support ended after a specified period of time; a lack of continuing support in some cases might account for difficulties in sustaining tenancies.
- Some services (such as the handyperson schemes) had some impact on improving the fabric of the housing.

The extent to which services enabled some people to remain in their own homes as opposed to a move to more institutional provision (such as residential care) was rarely measured, rather respondents intimated at the likely impact on retaining independence.

User-centred outcomes

A consistent finding across all types of service was that many users *felt* the service had added something to their life, particularly in helping them to feel more positive. Qualitative studies provided the best evidence of this: in the main, studies had not tried to measure such outcomes quantitatively.

- Qualitative interviews revealed that many users of low intensity services felt that their overall sense of well-being (including feelings of self-esteem, enhanced self-worth, confidence and attitude to life) had improved through being involved with the service. The effect, if anything, appeared to be stronger in more detailed qualitative studies.
- Other user-centred outcomes were evident including, users feeling more at home in their accommodation, feeling more comfortable and safer at home (particularly evident from direct practical services).

Social outcomes

A dichotomy was observed in the evidence of the value of social and emotional support. The importance of social support was universally stressed by users and service providers; however, while successes were observed from one-to-one relationships, there was little evidence that present services increased social activity more broadly.

- The relationship between volunteer and user is key to the success of a service: users derive a wide range of benefits from this relationship if it is not too time-constrained.
- Some housing/tenancy services had limited success in (prioritising and) addressing emotional and social needs, despite its central importance in sustaining tenancies.
- Most types of services (including befriending services) did not succeed in widening users' social networks – particularly when it involved meeting new people in the community outside of people with similar support needs. Further research is required in this area.
- Befriending and other services designed to address specifically the promotion of social networks sometimes have a low take-up by people with support needs and may therefore only be effective for some people.
- Few studies looked at the importance of support being delivered *by* users *for* other users; while mutual support schemes found there were limited, although important, outcomes from this type of service, it is clear that the potential for this type of support is under-explored in the literature.
- There was limited evidence of the *potential* value of virtual social support;
- No studies explicitly looked at the possible social and other benefits to users of finding employment or training (and rarely mentioned increased employment as an outcome in itself).

Health-related outcomes

While few studies looked at the effectiveness of services in improving health, available evidence indicated that services might expect to achieve significant outcomes in this area.

- A number of health gains were found from services aimed at people with specific health problems, including increased rate of remission for women experiencing depression and reduced drug use.
- Reduction in hospitalisation, inpatient use and so on were rarely adequately measured in studies. Examples of successes were given, but there was often a lack of information on prior health to measure the significance of the effect.
- In particular, some interventions led to users having an improved self-perceived health status (sometimes subjective measures showing a change when other, more 'objective' measures did not).

Wider community outcomes

Very few studies looked at the potential for low intensity support services to deliver wider social outcomes, for example on poverty and social cohesion.

- One study reported that service users were committing less serious crimes than before the intervention which would bring community gains (although the number of crimes had not reduced); and a possible reduction in the scale of local drugs market.

Towards a better evidence base

Overall, a higher priority needs to be placed on developing more robust sets of outcome measures for use in assessing the effectiveness of low intensity support services. The research community, policy makers, funders, service providers, and importantly, people with support needs, can all play an important part in this process.

Research community

The use of outcome measures in social care and policy research are still being developed (for example, a major project is currently being undertaken in the Social Policy Research Unit, University of York, funded by the DoH, looking at social care outcomes). The problematic nature of measuring outcomes in this field of study is acknowledged but needs wider debate. It is crucial that measures which are sensitive enough to assess the benefits of schemes are developed, rather than blunt tools which do not adequately measure the areas needed. Continued support to the research community is required to achieve this. Further, researchers need to be as open and honest as possible with each other in discussing the limitations of present research methods.

Users

At present there is no user involvement in developing outcome indicators. What do people receiving the services see as the main purpose and measures of success of a scheme? It is likely that user views in this area will differ from those of professionals and policy makers; older people placing a much higher value on domestic support, compared to professionals, is a clear example of this. It is crucial that the development of outcome measures involve users centrally in the process.

Research funders

Funders of research need to place a greater emphasis on outcomes in research specifications. However, they also need to be aware that there are likely to be cost and time implications involved in this. For example, studies may need to be conducted over longer periods of time to observe change over time, or, where possible, longitudinal studies may need to be conducted. Research with short time-scales may produce findings earlier, but ultimately, longer studies, if undertaken correctly, may produce findings which are more useful to policy makers, and users, in deciding which services to commission.

Service providers

Awareness of the importance of using sensitive outcome measures to evaluate services also needs to be heightened among service providers and practitioners. Commissioners and service providers need to be as explicit as possible about the aims of services, that is what they are trying to achieve. Routine collection of information by projects also needs to be improved, for example, collecting data on tenancy breakdowns.

Policy makers

Policy makers are already concerned with performance monitoring. It is possible that the new emphasis on measurement of outcomes in, for example, the new *Supporting people* arrangements, could lead to the collection of better information in this area. However, policy makers need to take a broader interest in the assessment of the effectiveness of services, and ideally help local authorities and other bodies to design better monitoring and evaluation of services. An opportunity exists for government to support social services departments in the monitoring of services funded through the new *Modernising social services* Prevention Grant. The availability of larger data sets in this area – something which would need to be supported by government – would also present better opportunities for examining effectiveness.

Finally, it is important that publications arising from studies on outcomes include more details on research methods. There appears to be a trend away from detailed description of methods in social research publications. With the proliferation of information in the area it is understandable that reports need to be concise; however, without an adequate description of methods, the task of assessing the quality of the research and, in turn, the robustness of the findings on outcomes, cannot be achieved. It is important that the undertaking of a systematic review is not the only time that research evidence is assessed for quality and consistency. All those interested in the development of better services leading to better outcomes for people with support needs need to become literate in the art of assessing research evidence.

References

Adam, S. (1992) *Taking the initiative: A study of the Home Improvement Agency Handyperson Service*, Nottingham: Care and Repair.

Age Concern (Scotland)/Engage (Scotland) (1999) *Volunteering from home: Telephone schemes and other opportunities for home-based people*, Age Concern/ Engage.

Andersson, L. (1998) 'Loneliness research and interventions: a review of the literature', *Ageing and Mental Health*, vol 2, no 4, pp 264-74.

Appleton, N. (1996) 'The value of handyperson's schemes for older people', *Housing Research Findings No 179*, May.

Audit Commission (1996) *Balancing the care equation: Progress with community care*, Community Care Bulletin No 3, London: HMSO.

Audit Commission (1998) *Home alone: The role of housing in community care*, London: Audit Commission.

Bayley, M. (1997) *What price friendship? Encouraging the relationships of people with learning disabilities*, Minehead: Hexagon Publishing.

Bowling, A. (1991) 'Social support and social networks: their relationship to the successful and unsuccessful survival of elderly people in the community', *Family Practice*, vol 8, no 1, pp 68-83.

Bradshaw, T. and Haddock, G. (1998) 'Is befriending by trained volunteers of value to people suffering from long-term mental illness?', *Journal of Advanced Nursing*, no 27, pp 713-20.

Burrows, R. (1997) *Contemporary patterns of residential mobility in relation to social housing in England*, York: Centre for Housing Policy, University of York.

Cahill, M. (1993) 'Computer technology and human services in the 90s: advancing theory and practice: teleshopping and social services in the United Kingdom', *Community Applications*, pp 231-45.

Clapham, D. and Franklin, B. (1994) *Housing management, community care and competitive tendering*, Coventry: Chartered Institute of Housing.

Clapham, D. and Franklin, B. (1995) *The housing management contribution to community care*, Glasgow: Centre for Housing Research and Urban Studies, University of Glasgow.

Clark, D.M. (1991) *Good neighbours: A practical guide to setting up a village care group*, York: Joseph Rowntree Foundation.

Clark, H., Dyer, S. and Horwood, J. (1998) *'That bit of help': The high value of low level preventative services for older people*, Bristol/York: The Policy Press/Joseph Rowntree Foundation.

Clarke, M., Clarke, S.J. and Jagger, C. (1992) 'Social intervention and the elderly: a randomised controlled trial', *American Journal of Epidemiology*, vol 136, no 12, pp 1517-23.

Cohen, S. and Willis, T. (1985) 'Stress, social support and the buffering hypothesis', *Psychological Bulletin*, no 98, pp 310-57.

Copello, A.G., Velleman, R.D.B. and Howling, V.M. (1998) 'The use of volunteers as befrienders within a community alcohol team', *Journal of Substance Misuse*, no 3, pp 189-99.

Crane, M. and Warnes, T. (1999) *Lancefield Street: Achievements and lessons*, Sheffield: Centre for Ageing and Rehabilitation Studies, University of Sheffield.

CVS Consultants (1997) *Feasibility study on floating support in Hampshire*, London: CVS.

CVS Consultants (1999) *An evaluation of HACT's Floating Support Programme: First Annual Report*, London: CVS.

Dane, K. (1998) *Making it last: A report on research into tenancy outcomes for rough sleepers*, London: Housing Services Agency.

Dant, T. and Deacon, A. (1989) *Hostels to homes? The rehousing of single homeless people*, Aldershot: Avebury.

Dean, J. and Goodlad, R. (1998) *Supporting community participation: The role and impact of befriending*, Brighton: Pavilion Publishing.

Deeks, J., Glanville, J. and Sheldon, T.A. (1996) *Undertaking systematic reviews of research on effectiveness: CRD guidelines for those carrying out or commissioning reviews*, York: NHS Centre for Reviews and Dissemination, University of York.

DoH (Department of Health) (1989) *Caring for people: Community care in the next decade and beyond*, Cm 849, London: HMSO.

DoH (1997a) *Community care statistics, 1996: Day and domiciliary personal social services for adults, England*, London: DoH.

DoH (1997b) *Community care statistics, 1997: Day and domiciliary personal social services for adults, England*, London: DoH.

DoH (1997c) *The new NHS: Modern, dependable*, London: The Stationery Office.

DoH (1998a) *Modernising social services: Promoting independence, improving protection, raising standards*, Cm 4169, London: The Stationery Office.

DoH (1998b) *Our healthier nation*, London: The Stationery Office.

Douglas, A., MacDonald, C. and Taylor, M. (1998) *Living independently with support: Service users' perspectives on 'floating' support*, Bristol/York: The Policy Press/ Joseph Rowntree Foundation.

DSS (Department of Social Security) (1998) *Supporting people: A new policy and funding framework for support services*, London: The Stationery Office.

Elsmore, K. (1996) *Being there: Tenants with mental health support needs: An analysis of working practices in London*, London: London Housing Unit.

England, J. (1998) *Evaluation of Capital Youth Link*, Unpublished report, Centre for Housing Policy, University of York.

Esmond, D. and Stewart, J. (1997) *Scope for fair housing (1): A literature review of housing with support for younger disabled people who require accessible housing*, London: Scope.

Franklin, B.J. (1996) 'Concierges in tower blocks: a strategy in the mediation of change', *Scandinavian Housing and Planning Research*, vol 13, pp 27-39.

Goldup, M. (1999) *An evaluation of five floating support schemes in North and Mid Hampshire*, Southampton: ROCC.

Goss, S. (1998) *A framework for housing with support: A tool to describe, evaluate and continuously improve services*, London: National Housing Federation.

Hall, J. (1997) *Survey of local authorities, 1996*, National Council of Domiciliary Care Services.

Hammond, T. and Wallace, P. (1992) (eds) *Housing for people who are severely mentally ill*, Kingston-upon-Thames: National Schizophrenia Fellowship.

Handyside, L. and Heyman, B. (1990) 'Community mental health care: clients' perceptions of services and an evaluation of a voluntary agency support scheme', *International Journal of Social Psychiatry*, vol 36, no 4, pp 280-90.

Harris, T., Brown, G.W. and Robinson, R. (1999a) 'Befriending as an intervention for chronic depression among women in an inner city: 2: role of fresh-start experiences and baseline psychological factors in remission from depression', *British Journal of Psychiatry*, vol 174, pp 225-32.

Harris, T., Brown, G.W. and Robinson, R. (1999b) 'Befriending as an intervention for chronic depression among women in an inner city: 1: randomised controlled trial', *British Journal of Psychiatry*, vol 174, pp 219-24.

House of Commons Health Committee (1994) *Better off in the community? The care of people who are seriously ill*, First Report of the Health Committee, vol 1, London: HMSO.

Jervis, M. (1988) 'Off the shelf scheme brings mutual benefits', *Social Work Today*, 23 June, pp 18-19.

Johnson, S. and Brooks, L. (1997) 'Sending in the paras', *Health Service Journal*, 11 September, pp 30-1.

Joseph Rowntree Foundation (1999) 'Low intensity support: preventing dependency', *Foundations*, January.

Kestenbaum, A. (1996) *Independent living: A review*, York: York Publishing Services.

Lee, M. (1994) *Drumchapel Elderly Homevisiting Scheme: Final evaluation report, 1987-1994*, Glasgow: The Volunteer Centre.

Lesley Andrews, C. (1998) *Housing management: Defining the boundaries*, London: The Housing Corporation.

Lewis, B. (1988) *Domiciliary services: A basis for discussion*, London: Cicely Northcote Trust.

London Housing Federation (1995) *Managing vulnerability: The challenge for managers of independent housing*, London: London Housing Federation.

London Housing Federation (1997) *The invisible tenant: How vulnerable tenants are disappearing in general need housing*, London: London Housing Federation.

McCullagh, A. and Rich, C. (1996) 'Local heroes', *Health Service Journal*, 14 March, p 37.

McIvor, G. and Taylor, M. (1994) *Making it out: Supported accommodation for ex-offenders – Identifying effective practice*, Stirling: Department of Applied Social Science, Stirling University.

Morris, J. (1995) *Housing and floating support: A review*, York: York Publishing Services.

Morrish, P. (1996) *Preventing homelessness: Supporting tenants with alcohol problems*, London: Shelter.

Muncer, S., Burrows, R., Pleace, N., Loader, B. and Nettleton, S. (2000) 'Births, deaths, sex and marriage ... but very few presents? A case study of social support in cyberspace', *Critical Public Health*, vol 18, no 1.

Murray, A., Shepherd, G., Onyett, S. and Muijen, M. (1997) *More than a friend: The role of support workers in community mental health services*, London: Sainsbury Centre for Mental Health.

Oakley, A., Rajan, L. and Turner, H. (1998) 'Evaluating parent support initiatives: lessons from two case studies', *Health and Social Care in the Community*, vol 6, no 5, pp 318-30.

Pettitt, G. and Frew, R. (1998) *Helping housing association tenants with support needs: Information gathering: A good practice guide*, London: London Research Centre.

Pleace, N. (1995) *Housing vulnerable single homeless people*, York: Centre for Housing Policy, University of York.

Pleace, N., Burrows, R., Loader, B., Muncer, S. and Nettleton, S. (forthcoming) 'On-line with the Friends of Bill W: social support and the Internet'.

Popay, J., Rogers, A. and Williams, G. (1998) 'Rationale and standards for the systematic review of qualitative literature in health services research', *Qualitative Health Research*, vol 8, no 3, pp 329-40.

Quilgars, D. (1998) *A life in the community: Home-Link: Supporting people with mental health problems in ordinary housing*, Bristol/York: The Policy Press/ Joseph Rowntree Foundation.

RADAR (Royal Association for Disability and Rehabilitation) (1992) *The right to a clean home: An initial report on the campaign by RADAR and Arthritis Care on the state of the home help service for disabled people*, London: RADAR/Arthritis Care.

Randall, G. and Brown, S. (1994a) *The Rough Sleepers Initiative: An evaluation*, London: HMSO.

Randall, G. and Brown, S. (1994b) *The move in experience: Research into the good practice in resettlement of homeless people*, London: Crisis.

Randall, G. and Brown, S. (1995) *Outreach and resettlement work with people sleeping rough*, London: DoE.

Randall, G. and Brown, S. (1996) *From street to home: An evaluation of Phase 2 of the Rough Sleepers Initiative*, London: The Stationery Office.

Randall, G. and Brown, S. (1999) *Homes for street homeless people: An evaluation of the Rough Sleepers Initiative*, Summary, London: DETR.

Rho Delta (1997) *Evaluation of the Mental Health Floating Support Scheme*, London: Rho Delta.

Salvage, A.V. (1998) *'Something to look forward to': A review of Age Concern visiting and befriending schemes*, London: Age Concern.

Sandham, J. (1998) *An evaluation of the Housing Support Project*, Warwick: Warwickshire Probation.

Schneider, J. (1992) 'Can friendship be fostered?', *Community Living*, vol 5, no 4, pp 14-15.

Short, C. (1993) *Good neighbours: A study of the contribution Good Neighbour Groups can make to community care in the County of Gloucestershire*, Occasional Paper 21, Cirencester: Centre for Rural Studies.

Simons, K. (1997) 'Getting a foot in the door: the strategic significance of supported living', *Tizard Learning Disability Review*, vol 3, no 2, pp 7-15.

Simons, K. (1998) *Living support networks: An evaluation of the services provided by KeyRing*, Brighton: Pavilion Publishing.

Simons, K. (1999) *The view from Arthur's Seat: A literature review of housing and support options 'beyond Scotland'*, Edinburgh: Scottish Executive.

Sinclair, I. and Williams, J. (1990) 'Domiciliary services', in I. Sinclair, R. Parker, D. Leat and J. Williams (eds) *The kaleidoscope of care: A review of research on welfare provision for elderly people*, London: HMSO.

SSI (Social Services Inspectorate) (1993) *Developing quality standards for home support services*, London: HMSO.

SSI (1999) *Promoting independence: Preventative strategies and support for older people*, London: DoH.

Thornton, P. (1992) *A positive response: Developing community alarm services for older people*, York: Joseph Rowntree Foundation.

Thornton, P. (1995) *The Homeshare Project: Report to the Community Care Trust of a study carried out by the Social Policy Research Unit*, York: Social Policy Research Unit, University of York.

Uchino, B.N., Uno, D. and Holt-Lunstand, J. (1999) 'Social support, psychological processes and health', *Current Directions in Psychological Science*, vol 18, no 5, pp 145-8.

Warner, L., Ford, R., Bagnall, S., Morgan, S., McDaid, C. and Mawhinney, S. (1998) *Down your street: Models of extended community support services for people with mental health problems*, London: Sainsbury Centre for Mental Health.

Widdowson, B. (1997) *Floating support: The Oxford model: an external evaluation*, Oxford: Connection.

Wray, M. (1996) *The work of the Housing Support Team: A monitoring and evaluation of its early months*, Unpublished report to the Department of Housing and Social Services, Haringey Council.

Yanetta, A., Third, H. and Anderson, I. (1999) *Evaluation of RSI in Scotland, interim evaluation*, Edinburgh: Scottish Executive.

York City Council (1997) *Report on the establishment and support service for City of York Council tenants*, Unpublished Housing Services Committee Report.

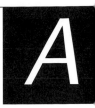

Appendix A: Sources of information

Databases searched

The following databases were searched in the review:

Social Sciences Citation Index

Via BIDS (Bath Information and Data Services). International multi-disciplinary index to 1,500 social science periodicals, plus social science articles from a further 3,000 journals. 1981 onwards. Updated weekly.
Records retrieved: 71

Sociological Abstracts

The major abstracting service for sociology and related disciplines, indexing over 2,500 journals worldwide, plus abstracts of conference papers, books and book reviews. 1963 onwards. Updated quarterly.
Records retrieved: 246

DH Data

Accessed via the Health Management Information Consortium (HMIC). Department of Health produced database.
Records retrieved: 382

King's Fund

Accessed via the Health Management Information
Consortium (HMIC). Database produced by the King's
Fund in London.
Records retrieved: 160

HELMIS (Nuffield Institute)

Accessed via the Health Management Information
Consortium (HMIC). Database produced by the Nuffield
Institute in Leeds.
Records retrieved: 144

Caredata

Database produced by the National Institute of Social
Work (NISW). Over 30,000 references to a wide range of
social work literature including government publications,
research reports and papers, monographs and journal
articles. Also includes JRF findings, NISW briefings. 1985
onwards. Updated quarterly.
Records retrieved: 200

ASSIA Plus (Applied Social Sciences Index and Abstracts)

Indexes and abstracts about 600 English language social
science journals, providing information on areas such as
social services, health, education, employment and race
relations. 1987 onwards. Updated quarterly.
Records retrieved: 78

Resline and allied databases

Database containing details of research projects and
associated documents on a number of related areas
including housing, urban and regional planning, local
government and policy services, construction and
transport. Produced jointly by the DETR and the London

Research Centre (LRC). Information collected annually from wide range of bodies undertaking research in these areas, including work being undertaken by the DETR. *Accompline* and *Urbaline*, the LRC's urban and social policy databases, were also searched at the same time, the latter particularly covering newspapers and press releases. There was a charge for these searches.

Records retrieved: 67 (Resline)
500+ (Accompline)
700 (Urbanline)

MEDLINE

The main abstracting service for the medical sciences. 1966 onwards. Updated monthly.
Records retrieved: 736

EMBASE

This database, produced by Elsevier Science, indexes more than 3,600 journals (and a small number of reports) covering the international literature on bio-medicine. 1980 onwards. Updated monthly.
Records retrieved: 383

PsychLIT

The leading databases for psychology and related disciplines, indexing approximately 1,300 journals, giving abstracts from 1987 onwards. Some book chapters and books also indexed.
Records retrieved: 495

CINAHL (Nursing and Allied Health)

Indexes and abstracts to over 650 international nursing and allied health journals, plus books/ book chapters. Since 1982. Updated monthly.
Records retrieved: 506

RCN Journals

The Royal College of Nursing database. 1985 onwards.
Records retrieved: 31

The Cochrane Library

The library presents the work of the Cochrane Collaboration concerned with evidence on the effects of health care interventions. It is held at the NHS Centre for Reviews and Dissemination, University of York. Databases searched within the library included the Cochrane Database of Systematic Reviews (CDSR) which gives full text of completed reviews and protocols undertaken by the Cochrane Collaboration, the Database of Abstracts of Reviews of Effectiveness (DARE) which provides information on previously completed reviews, and the Cochrane Controlled Clinical Trials Register (CCTR).
Records retrieved: 5 reviews
2 protocols (ongoing reviews)
18 Random Control Trial studies

SIGLE (System for Information on Grey Literature) and the Conference Paper Index

SIGLE is *the* source of grey literature for the UK produced by the British Library. There was a charge for the search: £114 for 110 records (title and so on, but no abstract). The Conference Paper Index was also searched at the same time but no additional records were retrieved.
Records retrieved 110

Hand-searches of library resources

The Joseph Rowntree Foundation and JB Morrell University of York library were both searched for relevant books, articles and research reports in the area of study. In addition, the small library holding of current housing trade magazines at the Centre for Housing Policy was also consulted. A number of newsletters or information bulletins were hand searched:

Signpost
DETR guide to research and statistics

The Bulletin
National Housing Federation

Link up
Newsletter of the Homelessness Services Unit

Prevention Works
Newsletter produced by Anchor Trust for the Preventative Task Group

Age Concern Information Bulletin
Monthly update on policy, practice and research

New Literature in Old Age
Centre for Policy and Ageing

Soundtrack
The newsletter of the National Development Team

OpenMind
The newsletter of the Mental Health Foundation

Campaign News
Newsletter updating the work of Scope's Campaigns and Research and Public Policy Departments

Internet searches

The websites of the following organisations were searched for both general policy background information on low intensity support services as well as publication lists of key studies in the area. In many cases, summaries of research studies could be retrieved directly from the websites, and occasionally the full text of reports.

Government departments and agencies

DETR	www.detr.gov.uk
DoH	www.doh.gov.uk
DSS	www.dss.gov.uk
Scottish Executive	www.scotland.gov.uk
The Housing Corporation	www.housingcorp.gov.uk
The Housing Corporation Innovation and Good Practice and Research database	helios.bre.co.uk/igp/
Scottish Homes	www.scot-homes.gov.uk
Tai Cymru	www.tc-hfw.gov.uk

Research organisations

Joseph Rowntree Foundation	www.jrf.org.uk
REGARD (database of ESRC research)	www.regard.ac.uk
London Research Centre	www.london-research.gov.uk
Norah Fry Research Centre	www.bris.ac.uk/Depts/NorahFry

Nuffield Institute for Health	www.leeds.ac.uk/nuffield/
PSSRU	www.ukc.ac.uk/pssru
Sainsbury Centre	www.sainsburycentre.org.uk
Housing Policy and Practice Unit, University of Stirling	www.stir.ac.uk/appsocsci/ housing/
Department of Urban Studies, University of Glasgow	www.gla.ac.uk/departments/ urbanstudies/
Centre for Urban and Regional Studies, University of Birmingham	www.bham.ac.uk/curs

Voluntary sector and allied organisations

National Housing Federation	www.housing.org.uk
The National Homeless Alliance	www.home-all.og.uk
Crisis	www.crisis.org.uk
Shelter	www.shelter.org.uk
Mental Health Foundation	www.mentalhealth.org.uk
National Development Team	www.ndt.org.uk
Scope	www.scope.org.uk
Care and Repair	www.careandrepair-england. org.uk
Age Concern	www.ace.org.uk
NACRO	www.nacro.org

Contact with key informants

Throughout the review, key researchers and policy players were contacted to check whether there was any new research in the area.

Appendix B: The search strategy

A search strategy was designed for use with all the electronically-based databases detailed in Appendix A. More information on the search strategy and review methodology is presented in Chapter 2.

1   support service*
2   support network*
3   support scheme*
4   support need*
5   support team*
6   support visit*
7   support* living
8   social support
9   community support
10 mutual support
11 living support
12 home support
13 care support
14 internet support
15 virtual support
16 virtual community care
17 supportive care
18 need* help
19 volunt* near support
20 housing management
21 home help*

22   informal help* or informal support
23   in-home assistance or home assistance
24   domiciliary service* or domestic support
25   resettlement near housing
26   special needs management allowance*
27   peripatetic warden*
28   practical advice or practical advice or practical support
29   support worker*
30   housing near support
31   community care near (housing or support)
32   non-professional help or non-professional support
33   untrained help or untrained support
34   unqualified help or unqualified support
35   supported housing or supported accommodation
36   #1 or #2 or #3 or #4 or #5 or #6 or #7 or #8 or #9 or #10 or #11 or #12 or #13 or #14 or #15 or 16 or #17 or #18 or #19 or #20 or #21 or #22 or #23 or #24 or #25 or #26 or #27 or #28 or #29 or #30 or #31 or #32 or #33 or #34 or #35
37   living skill*
38   run* a home
39   manag* a home
40   set* up home
41   day to day liv*
42   daily living
43   (bills or rent) near (pay or paid)
44   financial advice
45   money manag*
46   (complete* or fill*) near forms
47   (benefit* or grant*) near (entitle* or availab*)
48   cook* or clean* or decorat* or garden* or budgeting
49   shopping or laundry or ironing
50   household duties or housework
51   domestic tasks or domestic duties
52   meal prepar*

53 meals on wheels

54 healthy lifestyle

55 diet* advice or diet advis*

56 diy or handyman

57 advocacy or advocate or empowerment

58 access* near (services or facilities or resources or leisure or activities)

59 emotional support or reassurance

60 mental welfare or mental wellbeing

61 neighbours near relations*

62 social network*

63 tenan*

64 independen* skill*

65 liv* independent*

66 friend* or befriend*

67 (own life or own lives or own home*) near (run* or control* or responsib* or lead* or maintain* or keep* or remain* or stay* or sustain*)

68 #37 or #38 or #39 or #40 or #41 or #42 or #43 or #44 or #45 or #46 or #47 or #48 or #49 or #50 or #51 or #52 or #53 or #54 or #55 or #56 or #57 or #58 or #59 or #60 or #61 or #62 or #63 or #64 or #65 or #66 or #67

69 housing support

70 floating support

71 low* level support

72 low* intensity support

73 good neighbour*

74 (practical support) near (housing or home*)

75 (council housing or local authority housing or housing association or registered social landlord*) with support

76 keyring or home-link

77 (liv* independent*) near (housing or support)

78 domiciliary support

79 resettlement near (support or housing)

80   support worker* and (housing or home*)

81   (rehous* or re-hous* or resettl*) near (homeless* or excluded or isolated or vulnerable)

82   neighbourhood support unit*

83   community support worker*

84   preventative support

85   supported housing or supported accommodation

86   peripatetic warden

87   (ordinary housing or independent housing or general need* housing or independent accommodation) with support

88   resettlement near (rough sleeper initiative)

89   (housing manage*) near (support or health or community care)

90   support worker* and (housing or home* or community or team or tenancy)

91   tenan* near (support* or help)

92   #69 or #70 or #71 or #72 or #73 or #74 or #75 or #76 or #77 or #78 or #79 or #80 or #81 or #82 or #83 or #84 or #85 or #86 or #87 or #88 or #89 or #90 or #91

93   (#36 and #68) or #92

94   PY >= "1988"

95   #93 and (PY >= "1988")

96   CP = "UNITED-KINGDOM"

* 97   #95 and (CP = "UNITED-KINGDOM")

Appendix C: Data extraction sheet

Full reference:
Keywords:

1. Background to the study

- General background to study (funder; whether part of larger research initiative)
- Other relevant literature (note other main studies related to subject area)

2. Aims of the study (research questions)

- What are the precise research questions/aims of study and/or article?

3. Methods

- Quantitative, qualitative or mixed method
- Details on the sample(s):
  - size of sample (and population if relevant);
  - how sample selected;
  - whether any comparison groups;
  - characteristics of sample
- Location of fieldwork (both area and setting)
- Time-frame of study (dates; whether shap-shot or time series)
- Outcome measures (if any)
- Details on analysis, for example, if any statistical modelling

4. Main findings

Summary of main findings as they relate to the key review questions:

- What evidence exists that low intensity support services are effective in enabling vulnerable and socially excluded people to live independently?
  - In what ways are they effective? (Note measures used in the study)
- What makes low intensity support services (in)effective? (That is, what features of the service 'work'/do not 'work'?)

5. Overall evaluation of value and robustness of research

- Robustness of methods
  - Did they use the right methods to answer the research questions? (For example, should it have been qualitative instead of quantitative)
  - Was it a large enough sample/ purposive sample?
  - Were the response rates good or poor? (Might certain people have been more likely to respond to a survey or approach to be interviewed?)
  - Were any control or comparison groups used?
  - If qualitative methods used, how did the researcher illuminate the subjective meaning of those being researched?
- Internal validity of research
  - Could the findings be explained by factors other than the service intervention?
- Generalisability of findings
  - How far can the findings be generalised to other groups?
  - How far can the findings be related to the national context?

- Overall value of work
  - How up-to-date is the work?
  - Is this the first, only or best piece of work on this subject?
  - Is it national research?
  - Was the research undertaken by a reputable organisation (any possible bias?)

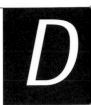

Appendix D: Summary of studies included in the review

Note: * The outcome resources were often *not* made explicit by the studies

Housing tenancy support

Category	Reference	Study	Main outcomes measures*	Key learning points
Floating support	Douglas et al (1998)	Exploration of user views	• User-centred • Social	• High level of satisfaction • Limited success in meeting social/emotional needs • Relationship between user and worker is key • Concern that support would float off
	CVS Consultants (1999)	Evaluation of HACT's floating support programme (first phase); mixed methods; national	• User-centred • Housing • Heath-related	• Varying levels of success at sustaining tenancies • Issues re support floating off • Support planning is key to the process
	Goldup (1999)	Evaluation of five schemes; different user groups; monitoring/ feedback questionnaire; Hampshire	• User-centred • Housing	• High demand for services

Rho Delta (1997)	Evaluation of pilot scheme; people with mental health problems; mixed methods (six user interviews); four London boroughs	• User-centred • Social	• High demand for services • Stability of tenancies • Importance of not rushing decision to move in
Widdowson (1997)	Evaluation of cross-tenure scheme; mixed user groups; mixed methods (five users);	• Recommendations of outcomes for the future	• Strategy for supporting people long term is required • Wider opportunities needed for users and members of the local community to become involved
Resettlement services Randall and Brown (1994a)	Evaluation of RSI1; homelessness people; monitoring/sample survey of 295 resettled people; London	• User-centred • Housing	• 40% did not receive enough help
Randall and Brown (1994b)	Evaluation of good practice by three resettlement agencies; homeless people; 117 questionnaires and 10 semi-structured user (and staff) interviews; London	• Housing • User-centred	• One third of users in rent arrears • Many users experienced loneliness

Category	Reference	Study	Main outcomes measures*	Key learning points
	Randall and Brown (1996)	Evaluation of RSI2; homeless people; monitoring/sample survey of 100 rehoused people; London	• User-centred • Housing	• 11% did not receive enough support • those not settled were younger, sharing, had few social contacts and were dissatisfied with the area
	Dane (1998)	Examined reasons for tenancy failure; RSI monitoring/quali interviews with 72 tenants; London	• User-centred • Housing • Health-related	• 16% failed tenancies – some more likely to fail than others • Multi-factors leading to failure, including social isolation, breif nature of support, health problems, etc
	Randall and Brown (1999)	Evaluation of RSI; homeless people; review of data; London	• User-centred • Housing	• Noted importance of resettlement plans, support from specialist staff, social networks and jobs/training
	Crane and Warnes (1999)	Evaluation of centre helping older homeless people resettle; London	• User-centred • Housing	• Older poeple and those homeless for shorter periods found it easier to resettle

	Study	Description	Type	Findings
	England (1998)	Evaluation of Capital Youth Link; young people; mixed methods; London	• User-centred • Housing	• Users wanted an open-ended service • Growth in confidence and living skills
Other housing support	Pleace (1995)	Support needs of statutory homeless single people; mixed methods four local authorities	• User-centred • Housing	• Importance of inter-agency working
	Elsmore (1996)	Review of practice of local authorities in supporting people with mental health problems; descriptive; London	n/a	• Highlighted partnership working
	Sandham (1998)	Support for drug users; case records (four users interviewed); Warwickshire/Coventry	• Health-related • Community • Housing	• Reduction in drug use achieved • Associated health gains • Less serious offences committed
	Morrish (1996)	Support for problem drinkers; five case studies; 26 interviews with drinkers; national	• Housing • Social	• Loneliness/social isolation a major factor in tenancy breakdown

Category	Reference	Study	Main outcomes measures*	Key learning points
	McIvor and Taylor (1994)	Supported accommodation for ex-offenders, including dispersed scheme; mixed methods; Scotland	• User-centred • Community	• Giving support and supervision together may negatively affect outcomes
	Warner et al (1998)	Five evaluations of a service for people with mental health problems; multi-methods including life skills and quality of life profiles and interviews; national	• Health-related	• Subjective assessments of health improved • Other outcomes more variable, but successes of reduction in patient bed use and functioning found in some schemes
	Handyside and Hayman (1990)	Impact of voluntary agency on mental health; circumstances and health questionnaire; control groups (three months)	• Health-related	• Improvement in health in both groups – three months not long enough to evaluate change?
	Murray et al (1997)	User views of value of support workers compared to key workers; 44 users	• User-centred	• Support workers seen as more available and more likely to understand needs • Emotional support important

Direct practical support

Category	Reference	Study	Main outcomes measures*	Key learning points
Housework and domestic services	Clark et al (1998)	Focus on older people's views; 51 interviews, consultation and key player interviews; three local authorities	• User-centred	• Highly valued, especially by women • Benefits: sense of control over life; enhanced self-worth; emotional/social contact • Relationship with worker key to success
Shopping	Jervis (1998)	Description of shopping scheme; delivered by people with learning difficulties, for older people; Liverpool	n/a	• Demand for service falls if charges introduced • Potential advantages: cheaper shopping; enhanced independence
	Cahill (1993)	Description of three tele-shopping services; mainly older people; two local authorities	n/a	• Potential advantages: enhanced independence

Category	Reference	Study	Main outcomes measures*	Key learning points
Handyperson schemes	Adam (1992)	Evaluation of one scheme; mainly older people; postal survey	• User-centred	• High level of satisfaction • Improvement in day-to-day living
	Appleton (1996)	National survey of schemes; also survey of users	• User-centred	• High level of satisfaction • Benefits: home easier to manage; safer; users felt mores positive; helping people stay at home?
Good neighbour schemes	Clark (1991)	Description of six schemes in rural areas; England	n/a	• Importance of good procedures/organisation structure
	Short (1993)	Survey of schemes in Gloucestershire; case studies	n/a	• Organisation of schemes is important
Concierges	Franklin (1996)	Examination of the role of 24-hour concierges; tower blocks; case studies; Glasgow	n/a	• Concierges appeared to provide flexible support to tenants 24 hours a day

Emotional and social support

Category	Reference	Study	Main outcomes measures*	Key learning points
Mutual support networks	Simons (1998)	Evaluation of KeyRing service; people with learning difficulties; quanlitative interviews including 49 with users plus attendance at tenants' meetings; London	• User-centred • Social • Housing	• Increased self-esteem • Enabled people to maintain tenancies • Importance of supporting relationships with neighbours • Examples of mutual support, altough downplayed by users
	Quilgars (1998)	Evaluation of Home-Link service; people with mental health problems; qualitative study including two rounds of interviews with 20 users; East Riding	• User-centred • Housing • Health-related • Social	• Ongoing contact valued • Increased confidence/ reduced anxiety • Enabled independent living • Varied impact on health status • Mutual support welcomed, but not everyone participated in networks

Category	Reference	Study	Main outcomes measures*	Key learning points
Befriending	Dean and Goodlad (1998)	National survey of schemes; six case studies including interviews with 28 users/31 volunteers	• User-centred • Social	• Problem finding volunteers and sometimes users • Benefits: companionship; ongoing contact; access to leisure opportunities • Limited evidence of broader social inclusion
	Harris et al (1999a, 1999b)	RCT; women with chronic depression (43 in study/control group); London	• Health-related	• Increased remission rate from depression
	Oakley et al (1998)	Operation of four Home-Start schemes; socially-isolated/low emotional well-being mothers; questionnaires to families; interviews with staff, four local authorities	• Social • User-centred	• Enhanced confidence for some • High proportion of families referred did not use the service

	Copello et al (1998)	Feasibility study based in a community alcohol team; feedback questionnaires from staff/volunteers and five users	• User-centred • Health-related	• Staff/volunteers thought networks improved more than users • Possible slight effect on drinking patterns
	Bradshaw and Haddock (1998)	Scheme for people with mental health problems; nine user interviews; Wigan	• User-centred • Social	• Improved self-confidence • Of the five people living alone, four did not see any change in social activity
Homevisiting	Salvage (1998)	Homevisiting schemes for older people; 20 schemes nationally; telephone interviews with scheme organisers	• Social	• Possible benefits: reducing isolation; prevention of moves into residential care; improved quality of life
	Lee (1994)	Description of Drumpchapel scheme	n/a	n/a
Telephone befriending	Age Concern (Scotland)/ Engage (Scotland) (1999)	Comparative study of four pilot schemes; support given by people who themselves have support needs	• Social • User-centred	• Value to housebound volunteers • Enhancing quality of life

Category	Reference	Study	Main outcomes measures*	Key learning points
Virtual social support	Pleace et al (forthcoming) Muncer et al (2000)	Exploration of Internet use by people with alcohol problems/depression/ disabled people; analysis of chatroom use/postings	• User-centred • Social	• User-led • Evidence of valued emotional/ social support and advice
Other	Clarke et al (1992)	RCT; 523 older people split into experimental and control groups; number of health and social measures; lay worker offered support aimed at enhanced social contacts; Leicestershire	• Health-related • User-centred • Services	• No significant differences in mortality, health, loneliness, social contact or demand for services • Experimental group showed improvements in self-perceived health status • Half the sample declined offers of health
	Thornton (1995)	Assessment of first 18 months of Homesharing scheme; older people; qualitative interviews (six users plus staff and volunteers); London and Liverpool	• Social • User-centred • Housing	• Older people in control • Feeling safer • Companionship valued • Helped people stay in their own home?